NUTRITION AND YOUR MIND

NUTRITION AND YOUR MIND

THE PSYCHOCHEMICAL RESPONSE

By George Watson

Foreword by W. D. Currier, M.D.

HARPER & ROW, PUBLISHERS

NEW YORK, EVANSTON, SAN FRANCISCO,

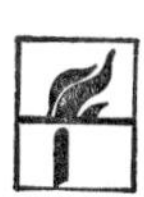

LONDON

1817

Reprinted with permission of author and publisher: Watson, G. "Differences in Intermediary Metabolism in Mental Illness," *Psychological Reports,* 1965, 17, 563–582, M2-V17. $1.00 per copy.

 For information address Harper & Row, Publishers, Inc., 49 East 33rd Street, New York, N.Y. 10016. Published simultaneously in Canada by Fitzhenry & Whiteside Limited, Toronto.

To Marilyn

Contents

Acknowledgments

Any continuing endeavor that spans two decades will inevitably engage the aid and support of a large number of persons, whether the ultimate issue of these efforts be ignominious or glorious. Those to whom I am so indebted are many, and I hope that all will know that I am indeed grateful for their interest and assistance.

I must acknowledge my special indebtedness to a few whose help in particular ways was essential to the completion of the research and this book upon which it is based: Dr. Elizabeth C. Bell and the William Bell Moore Foundation, Professor Charles E. Bures, Professor Andrew L. Comrey, Dr. W. D. Currier, and Gladys and Walter Lindberg. I would also like to express my deep appreciation to Mrs. Frances McCullough, my editor at Harper & Row, for her intelligence, interest, and perseverance.

Foreword

Emotionally disturbed people are perhaps the most difficult patients to treat. In order to give such patients at least temporary relief, doctors prescribe sedatives and other drugs—a treatment that may for a while ease the patient, but doesn't solve his problem. If the source of the trouble is truly a deep-seated or structural mental disorder, the doctor may not be qualified to tackle it. And a lot of investigation is needed before sending even the obvious candidate to a psychiatrist.

Freud, who invented the technique of psychoanalysis and is credited with "discovering" the unconscious, insisted that physical examination is the first step in treating emotional illness—a basic premise that was quickly forgotten in the flurry of enthusiasm for the new technique. Although psychiatry is now a highly developed field, very little of its expansion has been directed toward clarifying the physiological aspect of mental illness. In a sense, psychiatric treatment in the hands of rigid psychotherapists has been greatly responsible for holding back investigation and therapy in the field of the biochemistry of mental illness. Of course, psychiatrists have a vested interest, emotional and financial, in their particular field of practice, as do all other physicians.

Every function of the body involves a chemical process, whether it is physical or mental activity, even just breathing and feeling. When we get sick, we are suffering from a metabolic upset—a chemical imbalance. Ultimately, then, we must look to biochemistry for diagnosis and treatment. Sickness may attack only one small area of the body—maybe a cut on a finger—but many biochemical products are mobilized and carried by the blood to the traumatized spot to effect healing. The brain is especially susceptible to changes in body chemistry. And yet psychiatric diagnoses are almost always couched in terms which tell us nothing of the physical state of the patient.

Our willful ignorance about the sources of mental illness is not new. In the words of Henry Maudsley, a pioneering English psychiatrist, spoken in a lecture almost 100 years ago: "The observations and classifications of mental disorders has been so exclusively psychological that we have not realized the fact that they illustrate the same pathological principles as other diseases, are produced the same way, and must be investigated in the same spirit of positive research. Until this is done, I see no hope of improvement in our knowledge of them and no use in multiplying books about them." Apparently, Maudsley was right.

At present, the biochemical and nutritional aspects of mental illness are almost completely neglected. This newer approach to treatment, as suggested in this book, places in the hands of psychiatrists and other practitioners a tool of utmost importance. It is an addition to their own specialized knowledge and an indispensable adjunct to their modes of treatment. The more secure among them will approach this biochemical and nutritional therapy with an open mind. A whole new field of therapy may be his for managing one of the greatest medical problems on earth, the mentally ill patient.

Recently, some important studies have been devoted to the effects of deficiency diseases on mental states. In certain instances, retarded children have been found to suffer from a congenitally faulty metabolism in which a particular enzyme is absent or inactive. Even lay people recognize the manifestations of thyroid deficiency in their friends, such as lethargy and dullness, as well as the opposite personality traits of hyperthyroidism: anxiety, excitability, and nervousness. At last, the influence of nutritional deficiencies on psychic functions is beginning to be acknowledged. We now know that lack of vitamin B may lead to such serious diseases as pellagra and beriberi that can affect brain metabolism, producing symptoms of mental disorders. And starvation often brings about radical changes in personality.

Many of the mentally ill have inborn or acquired biochemical defects. Some adventurous psychotherapists are using what is called "mega-vitamin" therapy, such as the use of B-3 (nicotinic acid). Although this treatment helps many patients, it is oversimplified in using only one vitamin. Mental illness is often a manifestation of elaborately disordered metabolism, especially of the enzyme systems. Glucose metabolism, for instance, has a great influence on nerve tissue, which requires vastly more quantities of properly utilized blood sugar than any other tissue. Dr. Watson rather simply describes the extremely complicated biochemical processes involved.

It is dangerous to classify mentally disturbed persons solely in psychological terms. They may have the same symptom complex as others but for opposite biochemical reasons. In chemical testing, the norms for a mentally ill patient are not necessarily the norms for a mentally stable person. That is why, when chemical tests are run on patients with mental illness and compared with those for "normal" patients, they are frequently told, "There is nothing physically wrong with you. Go see a psychiatrist." Such a verdict is a cruel but accepted and medically ethical way of getting a troublesome, emotionally ill patient out of a physician's practice.

The old saying "You are what you eat" is not precisely true, although every function of the body, and especially mental activity, is dependent upon the quality and kind of food we eat, as Dr. Watson explains. Our genetic endowment plays a fundamental part in mental health, and some persons may become mentally disoriented when they eat or lack certain foods. Most people believe that they eat well-balanced meals, but routine dietary surveys show that there are frequently important deficiencies in necessary nutritional elements; this is particularly so in the mentally ill. The metabolic profiling Dr. Watson outlines can be used to advantage by any psychiatrist or psychologist to augment whatever technique of analysis or psychotherapy he routinely employs. I am sure that his own experiences will convince him of its value.

Mental health in general would be greatly advanced if every

physician and psychotherapist and every medical student would read this book. In addition to its direct application, some might be stimulated to enter the related research field, for—as with all knowledge—the surface has so far only been scratched.

W. D. CURRIER, M.D.

Editor's Note

Before making a self-diagnosis based on the suggestions George Watson makes, you should first check with your own physician. The science of psychochemistry is still in its infancy, and therefore many of the findings in this book come under the classification of theory–it is our hope that the publication of the book will spur further research and great public interest. In the meantime, it is essential to seek medical help in the treatment of psychochemical disturbances.

NUTRITION AND YOUR MIND

1 The Chaos of Psychotherapy

One day I received a phone call from a professor of classics I hadn't heard from in years. Professor McVay wanted advice on a distressing situation involving his wife.[1] Here is what he told me:

"The other evening Isabelle and I were watching television when, without a word, she got up and walked out the front door, down the driveway, into the street. I ran after her, calling, 'Isabelle! Isabelle!'

"She didn't seem to hear me. I caught up to her as she was about to step in front of an oncoming automobile. I grabbed her, and when I turned her around I saw tears streaming down her face. She wasn't able to say anything. She just kept turning her head slowly from side to side, and appeared to be gasping for air.

"I led her back into the house and she sank down on the couch and covered her face with her hands. I repeatedly asked her what the trouble was, but she only shook her head. I was frantic. My thoughts raced over everything that had occurred in the past weeks that might have upset her. But there was nothing I could think of.

"I thought a brandy might calm her down, so I poured some into a glass and added sugar and water. She began to sip it. Within a few minutes she seemed to be all right. Then she told me that at times during the past two weeks she had been overcome with dread. She felt a sense of 'impending doom,' a conviction that

[1] All names used in the case histories throughout this book are fictitious.

something terrible was going to happen. Yet at other times she was convinced that these fears were silly.

"I insisted that she see a doctor at once for a thorough examination, which she did. The results showed her to be in excellent health, except that her blood sugar was a little low."

Professor McVay asked whether I knew someone who could help Isabelle, someone she could talk to in order to find out the reasons for her attacks of panic.

"In the first place," I told him, "I really doubt that there are any 'reasons' for her attacks; and even if there were, I couldn't possibly recommend anyone. But let me arrange a consultation with the medical director of our research project. We have developed certain tests which might help spot the source of your wife's difficulties." The professor agreed.

A few days later I received a medical report on his wife. It showed just about what I had expected, based on his incidental remark that about a half-hour after sipping the brandy, mixed with sugar and water, his wife seemed perfectly all right—just as though nothing whatever were wrong with her.

To me this rapid recovery had only one explanation. Alcohol is quickly absorbed from the stomach and raises the blood sugar by acting on the liver to release glucose. Glucose is one of many kinds of sugar, but it is the principal fuel of the body. The brain and nervous system are almost totally dependent on it for normal functioning. Among the first things that happen if sufficient glucose is not available to the brain is loss of normal emotional control.

The report on Mrs. McVay showed that not only was her blood sugar barely at the minimum level necessary for her health, but in addition, her *oxidation rate*—our index for the speed with which her tissues were breaking down food to create energy—was far below normal by standards we had developed through our research.

We traced the two findings of low blood sugar and slow rate of energy production to a fad low-carbohydrate reducing diet she had recently adopted, which did not provide enough sugar to support the normal functioning of her nervous system. This appeared to be the sole cause of her attacks of panic; when we corrected her diet, the trouble disappeared.

After Mrs. McVay had recovered, her husband called to thank me for our help, and then he asked, "Would you mind telling me why you said you couldn't possibly recommend a psychiatrist or psychologist for Isabelle, supposing she might have needed one, since I know you work with some?"

Here is the answer to Professor McVay: Let us suppose that you have been feeling more tired than usual and are also having morning headaches along with other unwelcome pains in the chest and back that come and go without reason. You put it off as long as you can, but finally you call your doctor for an appointment.

After he examines you and has taken blood and urine tests, let us further suppose he suspects you may be developing a glandular disorder. He then tells you that it would be a good idea for you to see a specialist, an endocrinologist, and he gives you the names of several doctors, any one of whom—he says—can competently diagnose and treat your condition.

On the other hand, let us imagine that your doctor says he can find "nothing wrong" with you. This is, after all, about the most frequent result of investigating "vague" complaints. Now in this event your physician may think that your tiredness, headaches, and other pains may have an emotional basis. Does he now suggest you see a specialist, a psychotherapist, and does he accordingly give you a list of several, any one of whom is equally competent to diagnose and treat your condition?

No. He doesn't, because he can't. And he can't because there simply isn't sufficient *scientific* knowledge about the working of the mind upon which to base the art of psychotherapy.

Psychotherapy is a form of treatment practiced by psychiatrists (M.D.'s), clinical psychologists (Ph.D.'s), pastoral (minister) counselors, marriage counselors, and others without academic degrees who may call themselves "psychotherapists." The therapist tries to find the sources of the problem in order to change the thinking, feeling, and behavior of persons who are mentally and emotionally upset or ill. He does this primarily by listening to what the patient says and then interpreting what this means in terms of the underlying motives, attitudes, and beliefs of the patient. In simplest terms, the basic assumption behind this type of treatment is that the patient's illness results from unresolved conflicts, and their attendant motives, and attitudes. Further, it is assumed that when the patient becomes aware of his true situation, he will "see the light," so to speak, solve his hidden problems, and may consequently either recover from or adjust to his illness.

But just what is the basis upon which the psychotherapist determines which motives, which attitudes, and which beliefs are the causes of one's mental and emotional distress? How does the therapist determine precisely where the trouble lies?

Unlike the endocrinologist, who proceeds on the basis of factual knowledge of the glands and their functions in health and disease, the psychotherapist attempts to spot the causes of illness on the basis of principles and procedures that represent his own school of thought.

Schools of thought consist of different, and often contradictory, points of view. Needless to say, such divergent approaches to a single area of scientific investigation can exist only when factual knowledge is largely incomplete. There are no schools of thought in physics or chemistry, for example.

Unhappily this is not the case in psychotherapy, for here contradictions abound in the absence of concrete knowledge of the incredibly complex workings of the mind. What one practitioner may believe to be the causes of your trouble may be dismissed by another doctor bearing comparable credentials and practicing the same profession.

The reason your physician is unlikely to give you a list of several specialists in psychotherapy, any one of whom is equally competent to diagnose and to treat your condition, is that it is entirely possible that each therapist he might know and recommend might see in your condition an entirely different problem. Not just *one* problem, such as an overactive thyroid gland, which can easily and quickly be spotted by any endocrinologist anywhere in the world. Indeed, where psychotherapy is concerned, the nature of *your* "problem" depends almost solely upon the beliefs and practices of the therapist.

For example, a psychotherapist who calls himself a psychoanalyst and who also belongs to the Freudian school would probably interpret your headaches and other vague pains as neurotic symptoms which directly result from unconscious conflicts stemming from repressed sexual drives that originated in very early childhood. Now if your physician happened to send you to this practitioner, your "problem" is simply immense, for it may take years of treatment to resolve a long-standing "conflict" of this kind —if indeed a cure is ever achieved.

Another kind of psychotherapist calls himself a psychoanalyst but adheres to the Jungian school. He may flatly deny the Freudian interpretation. Since Jung did not believe that all neuroses could be traced to a single origin, but to at least three different kinds of sources, what the nature of your "problem" turns out to be in the mind of a Jungian analyst can't be guessed in advance. But the treatment probably will also be lengthy, and it will be entirely different from the one you might receive from a Freudian.

An Adlerian will look for unconscious conflicts involving feelings of inferiority together with desires for greater success and achievement. A follower of Otto Rank will dismiss what has happened to you in the past and concentrate on your present emotional relationships to see whether your family life, or your relationships with your employer, for example, are possibly upsetting you.

Or perhaps you might go to a practitioner who represents one of the newer schools of thought, such as Fromm's. If so, you may find the analysis of your "problem" is greatly simplified. Followers of Erich Fromm see all neurotic symptoms as evidences of a desire to escape from a precarious life situation, from the individual isolation and loneliness, the pain and uncertainties of existence, the inevitable specter of death. The Frommian will interpret your headaches and other vague symptoms as a technique you have adopted to avoid facing what to you is an intolerable life situation. Consequently treatment will consist of trying to change your basic attitudes toward life so that you feel more secure.

In addition to followers of Freud, Jung, Adler, and Fromm, there are of course many other schools of thought whose adherents call themselves psychoanalysts, and among whom the nature of your problem will reflect the nature of the beliefs held by the therapist.

Such divergent schools of thought could be enumerated almost endlessly. What these basic conflicts in belief and practice mean is that there is simply no foundation of scientific fact to support *all* of these contradictory schools of psychotherapeutic thought.

Each of the various competing psychotherapies claims to be effective as a method of treatment. This may seem incredible to the layman; to a scientist, it is not only illogical but also physically impossible. One's neurosis can't originate in infantile unconscious sex drives and at the same time definitely *not* originate in such drives.

In their book *How Psychiatry Helps* (p. 61) Dr. Philip Polatin, a Freudian "psychoanalyst" and his wife, Ellen G. Philtine, point out that many people are confused by the different schools of thought that have developed among psychoanalysts. Such differences of opinion, they claim, only confuse the outsider, not the therapist. And these authors conclude their chapter entitled "The Qualified Psychoanalyst" by saying that *any* psychoanalyst, regardless of the school of thought he follows, is equally qualified to help you!

Let us just consider some of the frightening implications of this claim. Suppose that you are suffering from an anxiety neurosis that really does stem from an unconscious conflict relating to infantile sex drives, as Freud believed neuroses do. Now, is every psychoanalyst equally qualified to help you? Suppose you consult a Jungian, a Frommian, a follower of Rank, Karen Horney, Harry Stack Sullivan, or a follower of any one of numerous other schools of analytic thought. Will his view of your problem and his treatment relieve your neurosis, even though he denies that infantile sex impulses have any bearing on your illness?

Well, if you share the belief of Dr. Polatin—which is fairly typical—the answer is yes.

This logic amounts to believing that although you ought to see an endocrinologist for the diagnosis and treatment of a thyroid disorder, you can be treated equally well by a dermatologist, even though he will ignore your thyroid gland and concentrate on a scaly scalp condition.

It seems that the "effective" part of psychotherapy is simply the act of visiting and talking to a therapist, regardless of what he believes to be the nature of your "problem." And as a matter of fact, there *is* a school of thought developed by Carl Rogers, which is based almost solely on this very idea that simply talking to *some-one* is "psychotherapy." In what Rogers calls "client-centered therapy" the physician listens to the patient's problems without trying to "interpret" what might be causing the mental and emotional symptoms. The most the therapist offers in this type of "treatment" is encouragement and reassurance to the patient that he can work out his own difficulties for himself *without* the help of the therapist! Sometimes this type of treatment, which consists basically of emotional support and encouragement, is called "supportive psychotherapy," and it is just about as far away from Freudian psychoanalysis as one can get. Yet these two incompatible schools of thought, occupying the very opposite ends of the psychiatric universe, are still called by the same name: psychotherapy.

Freudian analysis is considered even by its proponents as "the major surgery of psychotherapy." There are very few more mentally painful experiences than the emotional turmoil one can undergo during this kind of "treatment." Under just what conditions is such suffering warranted? Well, no one knows for sure, and many "psychoanalysts" deny that it is ever warranted.

The following case histories from my research files amply illustrate the seriousness of this problem to each and every one of us. For we all have a vital interest in the kind of medical care we may receive if we become ill.

A twenty-two-year-old unmarried woman volunteered as a research patient in a study of the effects of nutritional biochemical treatment in mental illness. Although she offered to participate in the tests, she did so rather reluctantly, urged by a friend who had personally witnessed some of the results we had obtained in an earlier experiment. The young woman frankly stated that she had no confidence whatever in the general physical approach we were taking to her kind of problem, but was convinced, rather, that she "needed psychoanalysis." When I asked her what she meant by "psychoanalysis," she seemed surprised that possibly I hadn't heard of it! I explained to her that the word had many meanings. She appeared puzzled, saying that she thought that "the standard treatment for mental disturbances was discovered by Sigmund Freud."

She gave the following information about herself in our initial interview:

She lived in her family home alone with her father. Her mother, a heart patient for many years, had died two years previously of a heart attack. She had two brothers, considerably older than herself. Her father was an excessively ambitious physician who had spent almost no time at all at home with his wife and children. If he took a vacation he went alone on a trip to a medical or scientific conference. Her recollections of childhood and early youth consisted mainly of painful memories of family arguments, of her mother having fainting spells and heart attacks as a consequence of such arguments. She felt her father had indirectly caused her mother's early death by his indifference, neglect, and cruelty.

She reported the following symptoms: severe depression with frequent suicidal urges; often she would stay in her room for days, afraid to see anyone; she developed an extreme revulsion for her father to the point of feeling like running and screaming at his sight; and she could not bear to have him approach her or touch her. She brooded over her mother's death constantly, and could not separate this event from her revulsion for her father. On the other hand, she would occasionally be overcome with remorse about her hatred for him and would admit to herself that she also loved and admired him.

Although she was convinced that the suggested biochemical treatment was "silly," she agreed to give it a fair trial. During the first month her worst symptoms began to disappear. Her depressed days became less and less frequent until they did not recur. And within three months' time she stated that she was well. Her attitude toward her father became normal. Six months after the start of treatment she became engaged, and she was married the following year.

This case is typical of those found in the literature of Freudian psychoanalysis, illustrating the theory of the unconscious origin of neurotic behavior owing to repressed sexual desires of an infantile nature. Here is an unmarried young woman, living alone with her father; she feels guilty about her mother's death and accuses her father; she is afraid to be near him, she both hates him and loves him, and she wants to commit suicide.

To a Freudian this young woman may have an Electra complex, in which the conflict between the infantile love of a little girl for her father, in competition with her mother, still continues unresolved in her unconscious mind, although she is now twenty-two years old. The psychoanalytic therapy indicated in such a case is to resolve this unconscious conflict, which, according to a practitioner of the Freudian school of thought, is the apparent cause of her abnormal mental and emotional behavior.

But was it actually the cause? Under treatment directed solely at improving the functional capacity of her brain and nervous system to produce energy, all of the alleged "symptoms of unconscious conflict" completely disappeared. Not one word was ever said to her in the context of psychotherapy. The amount of time that she had contact with the director of the research project was a total of an hour and a half—over a period of three months. In three thirty-minute interviews she was simply directed to take certain numbers of capsules a day and was given general advice on diet, to make certain that adequate fuel was available to maintain both her physical and psychological functions at an optimum level.

Now let us consider a different kind of case, one with a far less reassuring implication.

A thirty-year-old unmarried man presented himself to us as a potential research patient. In our initial interview he said that most of the time he felt a terrifying apprehension that something dreadful was going to happen to him, but he couldn't say what. During such an attack he was in a state of "almost unbearable panic" and felt that certainly he was "losing his mind." He could literally "see the walls closing in" on him, and felt that he was suffocating.

When I asked him about his previous treatment he said that he had been in Freudian analysis for a little over five years; for the first year he had visited the analyst five times a week, for the next two years he had gone four times a week, the following year his visits were down to three times a week, while the last year he went only twice a week.

When I asked him whether the treatment had helped him, he said no, that it had not only been ineffective, but that he was much more ill now than he had been at the start of his analysis. I then asked him whether or not he had told the psychotherapist that the treatment had made him no better but possibly worse. The young man said that he had indeed, and that the analyst had told him, "You are simply going to have to get hold of yourself–you are no longer a child."

During the first two months of our experiment this young man showed no improvement; nor did we expect any, for he was administered placebos (dummy pills) to see whether he might react to the suggestion that biochemical treatment was helping him. However, *one month* after the real treatment began he reported that his anxiety attacks appeared to have stopped, but that he couldn't believe it "after all those wasted years of analysis and no hope."

We observed this patient for about two years, during which time he remained psychologically normal, functioning in the community, and holding a job, none of which he had been able to do during his five years of psychotherapy.

These contrasting cases surely invite speculation on the ironies of fate. What if the young woman had received the Freudian treatment she really wanted and thought she needed, instead of the biochemical therapy she got? What about the young man, who was forced to relinquish a most promising career because of his anxiety attacks and spend five critical years of his life, those between the ages of twenty-five and thirty, in a futile, painful, and expensive venture into Freudian psychoanalysis?

Although we can only suggest speculative answers to these questions, we know certainly that in neither of these cases would therapy based on any school of psychotherapy have been appropriate. The young woman recovered completely without having to endure the ordeal of exploring this blind avenue. The young man was less fortunate, for he spent five years finding out that his anxiety attacks did not result from repressed homosexual impulses, as his Freudian analyst had supposed. Instead, his anxiety "neurosis" was directly due to the malfunctioning of certain mechanisms for the release of energy in his brain and nervous system.

I have not introduced these case histories merely to pronounce another negative judgment on psychotherapy. My object is principally to point out the kind of hazard one faces if he is referred to a psychotherapist for diagnosis and treatment of a supposed mental or emotional disturbance.

The words *psychotherapy* and *psychoanalyst* have so many meanings that they are virtually nonwords. The differences in diagnosis and treatment are staggering, and at this point the future course of your life may be determined by an accident of fate. For whether you spend five years or five months being "treated" depends entirely on whose hands you happen to fall into.

Why did the followers of Freud, such as Adler, Jung, and Rank, part ideological company with him? The simple and obvious reply is that Freud's ideas could not be checked out as being correct—as Newton's or Pavlov's could—by these men, who each then proceeded to try to do better. Ironically, none succeeded any better than Freud, for of these competing theories, not one has been able to win complete acceptance by students of psychology who themselves sought to check these alternate conceptions against their own observations.

The squabble leads us to a fundamental question: Is *any* psychotherapy really effective for mental illness? Controlled studies of the effectiveness of psychotherapies (including Freudian analysis) have shown that they simply are not an effective treatment for psychological disorders. Patients treated by these methods do not demonstrate that they improve any more than those who have received no treatment at all.[2] For example, Dr. H. J. Eysenck evaluated the results of nineteen studies on more than 7,000 patients and concluded that they failed to prove that psychotherapy—whatever the type—was of any value in helping patients recover from neuroses. He reports that roughly two-thirds of such patients will recover or improve to a marked extent within about two years of the onset of their illness, whether or not they are treated by means of psychotherapy (p. 125). In other words, while it is indeed true that persons undergoing psychotherapy sometimes improve, such improvement may be merely incidental to the passage of time. They could have improved equally well, as controlled comparative studies show, had they not been treated by psychotherapy at all.

[2] See A. Astin, *American Psychology* 16, 75 (1961); E. E. Levitt, *Behavior Research and Therapy,* 1, 45 (1963); H. J. Eysenck, *International Journal of Psychiatry* 1, 99 (1965).

This is one of the reasons why I declined to recommend a psychotherapist for Professor McVay's wife, Isabelle.

These negative assessments of the value of psychotherapy have come after almost a century of what now may appear to have been a vain endeavor on the part of a great number of gifted theorists such as Jung, Rank, Freud, Horney, and Sullivan. One can only wonder why it is that so many brilliant minds have been unable to penetrate the psychological maze that is presented by disturbed mental and emotional behavior. Can it be that the basic reason why all of these theorists have come to little agreement after almost a century of effort is because they have been looking for answers in the wrong place? The hard fact is that the most significant advance that has been made in controlling abnormal behavior has been through the use of chemotherapy rather than psychotherapy. Since the introduction of tranquilizers to American medical practice in 1954, the number of persons in mental hospitals has declined by more than 10 per cent while at the same time the number of persons requiring treatment has more than doubled.

This success of chemotherapy indicates that while contradictions may abound in psychology in the absence of real knowledge of the workings of the mind, we do, however, have real knowledge in some basic areas concerning the functioning of the brain and nervous system. And it is to this real knowledge that we must turn if we wish to understand the foundations of both normal and abnormal behavior.

The success of drug therapy in controlling abnormal mental and emotional states leads us back to the question of what causes such abnormal psychological reactions in the first place.

Suppose I were to give you a chemical (an antivitamin) that would block the utilization of the vitamin niacin in your central nervous system. The result would be "instant mental illness," most likely violence, during which you might smash all the furniture, throw it out the window, then run out into the street and attack and kill a total stranger passing by who had stopped to watch the ruckus.

In such an event your violent behavior would consist of "psychochemical responses"—not meaningful psychological ones.

Normal psychological actions mean something to the person

who does them in respect to his goals, desires, and wishes. In discussing another's behavior, for example, we say such things as: "I wonder why he would do that?" or "I can see very well why he did it." The actions reflect the person's intentions, conscious or subconscious.

But since psychochemical responses are merely reflections of disturbed brain function, they have no psychological meaning. Professor McVay's wife, Isabelle, who wandered out into the night, crying, presents a good example of such psychochemical behavior. Her actions had no meaning either for herself or for her husband, and resulted solely from impaired energy production in her nervous system.

The failure to distinguish between psychochemical behavior and motivated, meaningful behavior is at the bottom of the chaos in psychotherapy. For all of the competing schools base their theories and treatment procedures on the assumption that abnormal mental and emotional reactions are somehow deliberate and purposeful, and thus basically reflect the patient's "real motives."

The psychotherapists believe that such abnormal acts, in addition to having meaning, have been *learned,* either directly or indirectly, and thus can be *unlearned.* In fact, psychotherapy—regardless of the type—is basically an attempt to induce the patient to change his behavior, that is, to learn to act differently.

Now let us suppose that the abnormal behavior of a person such as Mrs. McVay really consists of meaningless psychochemical responses that are beyond her control, since they are caused by disturbed brain metabolism. Would her behavior change through "talking things over" with a psychotherapist?

Hardly. The only way to modify a psychochemical response is to correct the physical processes that are causing it.

In the case of Mrs. McVay, we changed her diet to raise her blood-sugar level and to increase the rate at which her brain turned glucose into energy. No amount of talking with anybody could achieve this result.

In our hypothetical example, in which an antivitamin blocked the brain's ability to use the vitamin niacin, resulting in psychotic behavior, it would be simply silly to search for psychological explanations for the murder of the stranger; the only remedy for this particular psychochemical behavior is to withdraw the offending drug and administer niacin so that the normal energy production of the nervous system can be re-established.

When we seek to understand the origins of disturbed behavior we must forget the idea that it makes psychological "sense." For it is this assumption that underlies all schools of psychotherapy, and it is this assumption that has proved fruitless both in helping us to understand abnormal behavior as well as fruitless in helping us to treat it.

Instead of trying to find the supposed underlying motives or "reasons" why persons behave abnormally, we must rather seek to understand what they do in terms of the biological malfunctioning of the organism. In general, abnormal reactions can be traced either to a structural failure—a hereditary defect such as a missing enzyme—or to a functional disturbance, which might be as simple as Mrs. McVay's low blood sugar, which resulted from a foolish reducing diet.

One of the main reasons psychotherapists tried to understand disturbed behavior strictly in mental, rather than in physical, terms was that early efforts to find physical causes were unsuccessful—though they go as far back as the medieval theory of "the humours." These early negative results led to the belief that mental disturbances were in no way linked to body disturbances, but were purely "mental phenomena."

This mentalistic assumption, coupled with the introduction of intriguing and mysterious concepts such as the "id," the "Oedipus complex," and "the collective unconscious," has had the effect of generating a romantic mystique in the popular mind concerning the origins of normal as well as abnormal behavior.

The creation of this fairyland aura around the psyche has also had the unfortunate result of hiding some of the basic facts of life concerning the physical foundations of behavior. Not only have these facts been obscured from the general public, but they also have been ignored by professional persons who ought to be better informed.

Many years ago a Freudian analyst asked me, "What on earth could nutritional biochemistry have to do with mental health?"

He asked this question after I had briefly mentioned some of the effects of semistarvation on personality which were revealed in a study conducted at the University of Minnesota. Since this therapist had never heard of the research, I described it to him briefly as being a six months' study of semistarvation undertaken by some thirty volunteer male subjects, all of whom were psychologically normal at the start of the test.

The semistarvation diet consisted of an average daily intake of about 1,600 calories, mainly carbohydrate, but including 50 grams of protein and 30 grams of fat. Even on this much food, however, which on the surface might not appear to represent a drastic deprivation, the group as a whole showed marked personality changes, both neurotic and psychotic. In fact, some subjects became so disturbed that they inflicted physical damage on themselves. One of the conclusions offered by the scientists who did this research was that "experimental neurosis" could be induced entirely by nutritional means. Since "nutritional means" are physical and not mental, the basic article of faith of all schools of psychotherapy—that minds must be treated with mental, not physical, techniques—is now in doubt.

From today's scientific vantage point, the concept of an independent mind is a carry-over from the speculative philosophy of the past. It has been replaced by the brain and the central and peripheral nervous systems—and by the internal chemical environment of the body in which all cells live and from which they obtain the materials that keep them alive and functioning. These materials are nutritional biochemicals, and they come from one and only one source: what you eat.

Consequently the answer to the question about how nutrition could possibly have anything to do with mental health is quite simple. What one eats, digests, and assimilates provides the energy-producing nutrients that the bloodstream carries to the brain. And any interference with the nutritional supply lines or with the energy-producing systems of the brain results in impaired functioning, which then may be called "poor mental health."

In the next chapter we will consider a wide variety of case histories which will illustrate how what you eat—and what you don't eat—directly affects your mind, your emotions, and the kind of person you are.

11 Psychochemical Responses in Everyday Life

John Gibson, an attorney I'd known for many years, asked me to have lunch with him. He wanted my opinion on something personal.

At lunch I learned that, after a dozen years of what he had believed was a happy marriage, he had recently discovered that his wife apparently didn't love him after all. In fact, it seemed to him that she hated him, and had for a long time.

I asked what led him to this conclusion, and he told me what had happened on his birthday: "It was late, around eleven, and Jan and I were sitting over coffee and an after-dinner drink. I pushed the drink aside because it didn't taste good to me. Jan looked at me with a puzzled expression. I said, 'I guess I'm just too tired to enjoy it'—and without reason or warning she shouted, '*You're* too tired!' And then she jumped up and ran to the fireplace, grabbed one of my golf trophies off the mantel, and threw it through the front window.

"I was terrified by the crashing sound of breaking glass and by the unexplained suddenness of her fury.

"'What's wrong? What have I done?' I managed to ask. But instead of answering she began shouting almost incoherently at me, accusing me of everything imaginable—selfishness, neglect, abuse—oh, I can't remember it all. She ran from the room, screaming and sobbing.

"I just sat. I was scared. In a moment she returned with her coat on and rushed out the front door, slamming it behind her. Just before she got into her car she yelled, 'Happy birthday!' and drove off.

"She came back several hours later, went to bed, and remained there most of the next day. When I returned from work I didn't mention the explosion. I later realized that she had no recollection of having thrown the golf trophy through the window, because she asked me how the window got broken!"

I asked him whether there had been an argument or some difference between them that had been building up to an explosion. But he assured me that he knew of nothing he had done that could have caused her violent reaction.

I had known Jan Gibson for many years, long before she married, and as far as I knew she was hardly the type one would expect to act violently. She was a thin, delicate girl, quite pretty and definitely shy.

I questioned her husband in detail about his wife's previous behavior, whether there had been other such outbursts or actions or moods that he considered unusual.

Indeed there had. He told me that he first noticed that something was wrong during a recent vacation trip they had taken to Central America. After the first week or so he realized that they weren't having their usual relaxed, enjoyable time together.

He said he found himself on the defensive day and night. His wife complained about almost everything he did or wanted to do: "Why do you have to dress so sloppy?" "Quit staring at the waitress!" "Can't you ever think of anything but eating?"

When they returned home, her petulance and nagging got worse. Nothing seemed to please her. The house suddenly had become almost unlivable in her eyes. To hear her complain, one would think the place was a shack. Some $75,000 shack!

But her principal target was her husband, and the outburst that occurred on the night of his birthday apparently reflected the tremendous amount of pent-up rage and smoldering hostility that she harbored against him. At any rate, this is how he interpreted her wild behavior. She simply hated him and could no longer hold it in.

To me, however, this conclusion seemed both simple-minded

and mistaken. Something else must have suddenly gone wrong. Two people don't live affectionately together for many years, as I knew they had, only to have one of them suddenly declare it all to have been a masquerade.

Consequently, I first questioned him carefully on one important point: Was he convinced that he first noticed the change in his wife's behavior while they were away on their vacation?

He said that he was absolutely certain of this, for he remembered what a good time they had together planning the trip. And even the first week they were away everything seemed normal. They had flown to New Orleans for a day, then on to Miami for several days before going to Central America. And it was there that their difficulties began.

He was obviously irritated by my line of questioning, for to him it seemed irrelevent. He became even more impatient when I wanted to know whether they drank bottled distilled water, and whether they ate raw fresh fruit and raw vegetables while in the tropics.

He said, "I know what you're thinking and you're wrong. We *didn't* get diarrhea or stomach upsets, even though we ate some raw fruit and vegetables. We also drank only bottled drinks. Really, my wife isn't physically ill!"

But when I asked him how they avoided the stomach and bowel infections that frequently attack tourists in the tropics, he said simply, "We just started taking sulfa drugs the minute we got off the plane—and that was all there was to it. We took them all the time we were there, and I think my wife is still taking small doses just to be sure."

"She *is?*" I asked, my tone of voice indicating my astonishment.

Sulfa drugs can inhibit the growth of bacteria: they are bacteriostatic agents. While taking such a drug it is possible to eat foods and drink liquids that contain otherwise harmful bacteria without suffering the usual stomach and bowel distress.

But there is another aspect of the use of bacteriostatic drugs such as sulfa or antibiotics that is definitely undesirable under any circumstance. They not only prevent the growth of *harmful* bacteria in the intestine—they prevent the growth of *all* bacteria, the good as well as the bad.

The normal "healthy" bacterial population of the bowel is called the intestinal flora, and its importance stems from the fact that the flora synthesizes a number of vitamins–such as riboflavin, biotin, and vitamin K–of great importance to the energy-producing activities of the tissues, particularly the nervous system.

For example, when the intestinal flora is not functioning normally, it is virtually impossible to substitute orally administered vitamins such as riboflavin that can adequately compensate for the lack of bacterial synthesis of these substances in the intestines.

We have also observed many abnormal psychological reactions in patients whose intestinal flora had been suppressed by drugs, or for any other reason, such as incorrect diet. These abnormal reactions include depression, anxiety, social withdrawal, irritability, and excitability–and a tendency to lose self-control.

That such abnormal psychological reactions indeed resulted from the suppression of the intestinal flora could be simply and dramatically demonstrated by administering a liquid culture of "healthy" bacteria–either yoghurt or acidophilus (a fermented liquid produced by growing *lactobacillus acidophilus* in milk)–preferably together with some starchy food such as bread or soda crackers, needed to supply the nourishment for the growth of the implanted bacteria. In most instances the abnormal psychological reactions would cease completely within a *few hours.*

As I began to discuss this subject my friend appeared skeptical and uninterested until I mentioned that mental depression was one of the first abnormal reactions that occurred when the intestinal flora was not functioning normally. He then told me that his wife had been "on the verge of tears" ever since they returned from the tropics, and that he had also been feeling very "low." However, he attributed his wife's depression as well as his own to the psychological conflicts that had recently occurred between them.

I told him that while it was clearly possible, however unlikely to my mind, that he and his wife were really at odds with each other, it was far more likely that their troubles were psychochemical rather than psychological, because of the unusual circumstances associated with his wife's recent personality changes.

At any rate, the simplest way to find out would be to check

whether or not their tissues were creating energy normally, and if not, whether intestinal flora replacement treatment would result in the expected psychological changes for the better.

When I talked to Jan Gibson the day she came to give us a blood sample, she confirmed what her husband had told me. She said that she had left home for their vacation feeling wonderful, but that everything "seemed to fall apart" during the trip. She also told me that since returning home she had felt so strange, so unlike herself, that she feared she was losing her mind.

Our tests soon revealed why she felt this way. Not only was her blood-sugar level too low, but the rate at which her tissues were turning food into energy—her oxidation rate—was about 30 per cent below normal.

This latter finding was surprising in view of the fact that Mrs. Gibson said she had stopped taking the sulfa drug at least two weeks before. Normally when one discontinues taking a drug that suppresses the intestinal flora, the bacterial population restores itself within a few days, *provided* one's diet contains sufficient carbohydrate—preferably starchy foods.

But since we also found that Mrs. Gibson's blood-sugar level was too low, this was evidence that something more than the suppression of her intestinal flora was contributing to her trouble—most likely her diet.

When I asked her about her food intake, she told me that she had gained several pounds while on vacation. When she returned home she decided to reduce by eliminating virtually *all* carbohydrates! She had picked up a book at the airport newsstand about a "low-carbohydrate diet," and what it recommended seemed so easy to follow that she began dieting as soon as she returned home.

Three days after our interview she telephoned and said, "Thank God. I am beginning to feel like Jan Gibson again."

She had followed my suggestion that she change her diet to include adequate calories from carbohydrates, including starchy foods, and in addition, to take yoghurt or acidophilus until she felt normal psychologically.

This case gives us an excellent illustration of behavior that simply has no psychological meaning, since it resulted solely from abnormal body chemistry. It also points up the fact that it is not only a foolish mistake, but also it may be downright dangerous, always to try to make psychological "sense" out of another's behavior, particularly when that behavior is not typical of the person performing it. In this instance, John Gibson was about to make a very serious mistake—one that could have led to a broken marriage.

The source of all the energy expended by the mind—considered as the function of the brain—is provided by a process called "cellular respiration," during which complex foods are broken down into simpler substances which are then burned (oxidized) in the individual cells of the brain.

The principal fuel of the brain is glucose, a simple type of sugar. This is the material that is carried in the blood, the so-called blood sugar, to all of the body's vital tissues such as the heart, liver, muscles, and brain.

Although glucose can be obtained directly from some foods, such as honey and grapes, the body manufactures most of its requirements from other carbohydrates (potatoes, bread, cereals), milk sugar (lactose), fruit sugar (fructose), as well as from meat and other protein foods.

In addition to glucose, many cells of the body can also burn fat for energy, even though it is not the fuel they prefer. The brain, however, appears to rely heavily on glucose for its energy, and, unlike other organs, it cannot switch to burning fat when sugar isn't available.

To illustrate just how important the sugar supply carried by the blood to the brain is, let us consider some of the immediate psychological effects that result when this supply is diminished.

Among the first things that happen when the blood sugar is too low and sufficient glucose is not available to the brain is loss of normal emotional control. This can take many forms, from simple nervousness, unexplained weeping and depression, all the way to violent impulses, the immediate urge to smash something—*anything*—just as Jan Gibson did.

These drastic emotional consequences resulting from impaired brain function are due to a combination of factors. First, the brain derives most of its energy from glucose; second, it cannot switch to burning other fuel when sugar supplies are low; and third, the brain consumes up to 25 per cent of the total amount of glucose carried by the blood, even though the brain accounts for just a tiny fraction (2½ per cent) of the total weight of the body.

Although normal brain function depends on getting enough sugar, this involves considerably more than merely eating something like honey which supplies glucose. For under certain conditions, sugar alone may *lower* the blood-sugar level. In fact, the problem of eating properly to ensure a constant supply of glucose for the blood is quite complicated. We will consider this question more fully later.

Under normal conditions the blood-sugar level is directly maintained by two different types of food: carbohydrates (starches and sugars) and protein (from meat, fish, eggs, milk products, and some vegetables and cereals). The blood-sugar level is also indirectly influenced by the amount of fat being burned in the tissues.

While all of the carbohydrates one eats are transformed into glucose, only about half of the protein in the diet can be transformed into blood sugar.

Even though the sugar carried in the blood is the principal source of energy of the body, including the nervous system, very little of this critically important substance can be stored for later use. A person weighing 115 pounds stores only enough sugar to last about four hours.

The principal storage site is the liver, where it is stored as "liver sugar" (glycogen). And it is in this form of liver sugar that part of the protein foods one eats contributes to helping maintain a normal blood-sugar level. Protein is first converted to glycogen (liver sugar), and then to glucose (blood sugar), by a process which is called gluconeogenesis.

Here is a brief summary of how the blood-sugar level is directly maintained: When one eats a balanced meal, the carbohydrate is quickly digested and transformed into glucose. Part of the glucose is carried by the blood circulating to the tissues for fuel, while some is stored in the liver as glycogen.

Protein, however, is much more slowly digested, and that portion which is capable of being transformed into glycogen is gradually stored between meals in the liver, and is then released into the blood as glucose when needed.

Consequently when the sugar in the blood that has been derived from carbohydrate begins to be depleted, there will be a reserve supply available from protein, provided the food intake contains adequate carbohydrate in addition to protein.

The reason why protein alone cannot contribute to the liver's store of glycogen and therefore to the sugar in the blood is that there is an interlocking dependence between carbohydrate and the capability of the tissues to transform protein into blood sugar. Unless sugar is being burned, protein cannot be converted into either liver sugar or blood sugar.

In the light of these considerations about some of the relationships between food intake and the blood-sugar level, let us take another look at the case of Jan Gibson, and examine a little more closely some of the biochemical reasons for her emotional explosion on the night of her husband's birthday.

Not only was Mrs. Gibson's blood-sugar level far too low, but the rate at which her tissues were turning food into energy was 30 per cent below normal. Since a low blood-sugar level at once implicates one's diet, I first questioned Mrs. Gibson about her food intake, and she told me she was following a low-carbohydrate diet.

You have probably heard about this low-starch, low-sugar way to lose weight that appears to defy the laws of nature. This approach to dieting allows one to consume practically all the *calories* one desires, just as long as these units of food energy come from protein, fat, or alcohol. The only concern one need have in counting calories is to restrict those that come from carbohydrates. And the upper daily limit that is allowed in the way of fruit, bread, or starchy vegetables like potatoes is about 2 ounces (60 grams), which yield about 246 calories.

Now suppose that you are a thirty-year-old woman, like Jan Gibson, and you weigh 128 pounds. The recommended daily food intake for you is 2,300 calories. Your brain alone will need 500 calories of carbohydrate a day!

On the low-carbohydrate diet, in which the maximum allowance of foods which the body can directly utilize to make sugar is only *one-half* of what the brain alone requires, the results can be disastrous. Not only will the brain be severely deprived of glucose, but the extreme restriction of carbohydrate will prevent the tissues from converting protein into sugar. And unless this latter process is functioning normally, it is literally impossible to maintain a normal blood-sugar level.

While it is true, as I pointed out earlier, that up to 50 per cent of the protein consumed in a balanced diet can contribute to the sugar stores in the liver and can help maintain the blood-sugar level, this whole system of converting protein to sugar fails in the absence of adequate amounts of carbohydrate in the diet.

In the light of these considerations one can see that the total effect of the low-carbohydrate diet that Mrs. Gibson decided to try was similar to starvation, during which the body doesn't have access to carbohydrates and must rely on burning its own stores of fat. The body cannot maintain a normal blood-sugar level. This is part of the reason why we found that Mrs. Gibson's oxidation rate was 30 per cent below normal.

Since Mrs. Gibson was virtually starving—unknowingly, for she kept eating—her emotional disturbance shouldn't really be surprising. For abnormal psychological reactions always accompany any dietary restriction of nutrients necessary to maintain the normal energy-producing capabilities of the central nervous system. Such personality changes are not always as obvious as Jan Gibson's, for often they involve actions which on the surface may appear to reflect rational behavior.

One of the subtler and really ominous types of psychochemical reactions that one sees when essential foods such as sugar and starch are severely restricted in the diet is an alienation from others, a suspicion and distrust of even those who have been closest to you. These paranoid reactions have been universally noted in studies of starvation and of even partial food deprivation, and they result directly from the inability of the brain and nervous system to produce their normal level of energy.

Although carbohydrates play an indispensable role here, their importance is nevertheless relative. For neither a normal blood-sugar level nor an optimum production of energy in the central nervous system can be maintained on a *high*-carbohydrate diet—

one that consists principally of fruit, cereals, and starchy vegetables.

In fact, such a high-carbohydrate diet is every bit as hazardous psychologically as the low-carbohydrate diet we have just considered.

We studied an interesting eighteen-year-old girl who, in describing herself as a "mental case," said that every morning she had to "crank up her courage to face the world." She was getting more afraid of everything all the time. When I asked her to tell me a little more concretely what she was afraid of, she told me that she hardly knew where to begin.

"I'm afraid of glass doors and big glass windows, stairways, elevators, bridges—they really *do* collapse, you know—tunnels, traffic, germs, letters." She stopped, out of breath, and then added, "I really mean I'm just about afraid of *everything,* like I said."

What puzzled her about this was that she never used to be afraid of anything or anybody. She had been socially and athletically active in high school. It appeared to her that these vague fears had begun several months after she graduated from school and took a job as a trainee in the telephone company. She said she first recognized that something was wrong when she found herself crossing the street to avoid meeting people that she had once been quite friendly with.

Our blood tests indicated to us that her tissues were relying disproportionately on carbohydrate for energy. In addition, her fasting blood-sugar level was minimal, and the total lipids (fats) in her blood were also unusually low.

To check the most likely source of these findings—her diet—we asked her to make a record of everything she ate for a period of one week.

Here is what turned out to be a typical day's food intake for her:

Breakfast: doughnut or sweet roll
black coffee

Lunch: mashed potatoes and gravy
green salad with vinegar dressing
coconut pie
Coke

Dinner: green salad with oil dressing
small serving of meat or fish
potatoes or rice
two other vegetables, such as carrots, beets, or peas
pie, cake, or ice cream
milk

This food selection represents a very high starch and sugar intake, and a very low protein and fat intake.

Detailed questioning revealed that this strange eating pattern was *not* typical of her meals before she obtained her job and before she developed her fears.

When going to school, she ate a regular "juice, bacon and egg, toast, milk" breakfast with the family. Now she had to get up too early to eat at home. She often barely caught the bus to work, allowing just a few spare minutes to "grab something" at the cafeteria before going to her office.

She ate lunch at the company cafeteria, and took what "tasted best," without knowing any better. On the other hand, when going to school, her mother always packed her a substantial lunch—meat or cheese sandwiches, milk and fruit.

The fact that she ate a fair dinner at home was her only nutritional safeguard, and it alone was not enough to meet the needs of her nervous system.

Earlier it was pointed out that the blood-sugar level is directly maintained by the carbohydrates in the diet, backed up by the sugar reserves stored in the liver, which have been derived from protein. In addition to these direct sources of blood sugar, the fat in the diet (such as butter and the fat contained in meat) indirectly influences the level of sugar in the blood.

In order to understand why this is so, it is necessary to consider briefly some of the main ways the cells derive energy from food.

Although it is customary to speak of the oxidation, or burning, of glucose, this is not a direct process. Glucose, as well as other fuels, is transformed into a series of intermediate compounds in an interlocking, step-by-step process, during which energy is formed. In other words, energy is not derived directly from glucose, but from several different substances, called "intermediates," each of which ultimately has been derived from glucose. The most important of these is acetate (acetyl coenzyme A), from which about 80 per cent of the energy produced in the cells is derived.

It is of considerable practical importance to recognize that virtually all foods—starch, sugar, protein, fat, and even alcohol—are transformed into acetate; it is the chemical transformation of this compound that provides the principal source of energy in the cells.

The richest source of acetate is fat, which proportionally yields more than three times more of this substance than does sugar, and up to about twice that derived from protein (depending on its type). And although the liver is the principal organ for transforming fat to acetate, this compound leaves the liver (in a chemically different form) and enters what is called the metabolic pool, the bloodstream, by which it is carried to other tissues, including the brain, where it can be transformed into energy.

Thus, while the brain primarily breaks down glucose and has very little ability to burn fat, it can, on the other hand, use the energy-rich intermediate acetate, formed from other fuels in other tissues, such as the liver. In other words, the energy-producing capability of the nervous system is affected by what is going on in other parts of the body.

However, the brain's ability to transform acetate into energy depends on the availability of other substances which are provided principally by the oxidation of sugar. That is, there is an interlocking dependence between the burning of glucose and the transformation of acetate into energy. This important point we will return to later when we discuss how an unbalanced diet can adversely affect the mind and the emotions.

Since about 80 per cent of the energy created in the tissues comes from acetate, you can see that if it were possible to directly measure the level of this compound in the cells, we would possess a much clearer idea of the energy-producing potential of the tissues than we now do. At present we must rely on indirect tests.

One of these tests, of course, is the blood-sugar level. If this is very low, acetate—even if available—cannot be turned into energy, since it is the breakdown of sugar which supplies the biochemical means by which energy may be derived from acetate.

Another indirect index of the cellular acetate level is the total fat content of the blood, for when this is very low, the richest source of acetate is limited.

In order to better understand the practical implications of these considerations, let us take another look at our fearful young lady.

In psychological terms we would say that she "lacked ego strength"—that is, she possessed no confidence, no courage, and was literally afraid of everything. And as you may recall, our laboratory tests indicated that she was relying largely on starch and sugar for energy.

In addition, we had found that both her blood-sugar level and her blood-fat level were very low.

If we now translate these findings into an estimate of the amount of energy being produced in her nervous system, we must conclude that it was low indeed. Her high-carbohydrate diet was inadequate to maintain a normal blood-sugar level, partly because she was not getting enough protein to maintain a reserve supply of stored sugar (glycogen) in the liver.

In addition, her fat intake was insignificant, which also has a bearing on her low blood-sugar level. For in the absence of acetate derived from fat, the cells quickly exhaust the small amount of acetate that the blood sugar alone can supply, and this is not enough to provide for the optimum functioning of the cells.

In this case, if we use the phrase *acetate level* to refer to the potential energy-producing capability of the tissues, we see that her high-carbohydrate, low-fat, low-protein diet simply did not provide a sufficient amount of this energy-rich intermediate to provide her with the mental and emotional strength she formerly possessed.

Since she was young and healthy, however, and had not been on this poor diet long enough to cause any significant damage to her enzyme systems—that is, her capacity for turning food into energy—she recovered from being what she herself had described as a mental case within a few weeks after being advised to change her eating pattern.

Her fears disappeared, her confidence reasserted itself, and she found herself actually crossing the street to say hello to a friend, rather than crossing the street to avoid one.

This case had a simple and happy resolution, mainly because the source of trouble was discovered soon enough, before any damage had been done to the energy-producing systems in the cells. More often, however, one encounters problems whose resolutions are not quite so easy.

For example, we studied a young man suffering from mental depression accompanied by severe claustrophobia (a morbid fear of small enclosures). He had been unable to take a bath or shower for more than five years! He simply could not remain in a bathroom long enough to shower before he would be overcome by sheer panic.

Our tests indicated that he was unable to break down glucose normally, and consequently was unable to derive the major part of energy available to the cells from acetate.

His dietary history was peculiar indeed: He ate only hamburger, or so he said, "balanced" by coffee with skim milk. (He also smoked cigarettes incessantly–*both* his hands were stained yellow.)

When he described this diet to me I simply couldn't believe it. But when I asked his mother about it, she said, "Yes, Donald really loves his hamburger."

I questioned Donald about his unusual eating practices, expressing alarm and dismay that anyone would so abuse his mind and body. He became quite hostile and defensive and demanded, "What's wrong with hamburger?"

Now, although there is obviously nothing "wrong" with hamburger, there is everything wrong with eating *only* hamburger, or eating *only* anything else, for that matter. Here is why:

Earlier I indicated that energy is released in the cells by a series of interlocking chemical reactions. Each of these reactions requires the participation of a specific enzyme.

In one respect enzymes may be likened to the spark plugs in an automobile engine; without them the engine won't run. Similarly, the biochemical reactions on which the release of energy depends simply do not take place without enzymes. In one important respect, however, enzymes differ from spark plugs; enzymes must be regenerated—renewed continually, they are not designed to last for 20,000 miles.

The materials required for the continuous renewal of enzymes come from only one source: the food one eats. Although the complexities of this subject need not concern us here, for there are hundreds of enzymes in the body, it is important to point out that the proper maintenance of the various enzyme systems requires a continuous supply of a wide range of nutritional substances (including especially vitamins and minerals).

This is why a diet of hamburger and coffee, or a limited and unvarying diet of any kind, can result in literally wrecking the energy-producing systems of the body. And there is no "perfect" food, no "perfect combination" of foods, that can be relied on to provide all of the nutrients one needs under any and all circumstances.

As for the young man who had been living for several years on hamburger and coffee, we found that his tissues had all but lost their capacity to convert food into energy. When he was placed on a diet containing adequate carbohydrate, fat, and protein, and including fruit and vegetables that normally supply some of the essential vitamins and minerals that the body requires for the renewal of enzymes, we found that he was still unable to utilize these nutrients normally.

However, when he was given large quantities of certain vitamins and minerals he had been missing on his hamburger diet, he gradually improved, over a long period of time, and as his ability to produce energy improved, his depression and fears left. He regained the ability to remain in a small enclosure without panic.

Each of these case histories illustrates a kind of psychochemical response that results from a diet that is in some vital way inadequate to support the normal operation of the brain and nervous system.

In addition to the role that one's food intake may play in adversely affecting mood, emotion, and behavior, there are many other factors besides diet that also may cause psychochemical responses.

Several years ago I invited a professor friend and his wife to a small gathering. Professor Gerald Hunt was a psychologist, and although he had a Freudian approach, he also had scientific caution and an open mind. Because of this we found common ground; for despite his tendency to try to make Freudian "psychological sense" out of each and every thought, word, or deed, he was most interested in my biochemical approach to behavior and had given me help and encouragement over the many years we had known each other.

Dr. Hunt said he would very much like to attend our party, but that his wife wasn't feeling well enough to go out. When I told him that I was sorry to hear she was ill, he said that she wasn't "ill" in that sense at all.

"Janet is just going through her usual holiday blues," he said, "although for some reason they've hit her a lot sooner this year than usual."

I privately reacted both quickly and negatively to this "holiday blues" idea—to the notion that his wife had learned, through long and sad experience, that the Christmas holidays were a time of grief.

I asked him what he believed to be the cause of his wife's depression at the approach of Christmas each year.

"Well," he began, defensively adopting the lecture-hall tone of authority, "this of course extends way back to her early childhood, and obviously involves her formative relationships with her parents. . . ."

He talked on in this vague psychoanalytical vein for some time without my saying anything, until he made the remark, "One thing I can't figure out is that some years she really *enjoys* Christmas and the holidays. Last year, for example, she was very happy during the Christmas season, and we even held a small party, as you probably remember. I thought at the time that possibly she was growing up emotionally, and overcoming some of her infantile reactions."

This line of thinking, vague and inconsistent, irritated me considerably.

I said, "Look, Gerry, do you really believe all that junk you just told me about your wife's repressed unconscious infantile conflicts as being the cause of her 'holiday blues'? Particularly when some years she really looks forward to Christmas and has a very good time?"

Blunt, and possibly a little brutal, but I saw no reason why his wife should continue to suffer for *his* psychological misconceptions, and I told him so.

I also pointed out that since his wife apparently did not *dislike* the Christmas season as such, some factors other than psychological ones must be affecting her adversely. I suggested that he let us explore the matter from our psychochemical point of view.

After a brief, face-saving conversation, he hesitantly agreed to ask his wife to volunteer to become one of our research patients.

It had been an unusually cold winter in Pasadena, and it was actually snowing a little the morning Janet Hunt arrived for her initial interview. The first thing she said was, "I'm freezing on the *inside,* and have been for weeks!" She said she simply couldn't get warm, even though she kept the thermostat in their apartment set at eighty degrees. As she told me this she appeared to be shivering, her hands trembling in that involuntary muscular activity the body sets in motion to create warmth when the tissues aren't producing sufficient heat.

Since Mrs. Hunt was visibly cold, and because most of the heat produced in the body results from the oxidation of fuel in the tissues, it was obvious to me that she was not at that moment creating sufficient energy to compensate for the loss of body heat to the cold air around her. Since the main sources of heat in the body are the most active tissues, which include the brain, one would have to expect that this important organ was also "feeling the effect" of the cold. There would be a lowered level of functioning owing to the loss of energy as heat.

Our blood tests indicated why Mrs. Hunt was "freezing on the inside." Although her blood-sugar level was in the low-normal range, the total fat concentration in her blood, an indirect indicator of her cellular acetate level, was but one-half of what it should have been.

As we mentioned earlier, about 80 per cent of the oxidative energy in the tissues results from the breakdown of acetate, and dietary fat is the most concentrated source of this energy-rich intermediate. This is why high-fat diets have been found to be superior in helping maintain normal body temperature in cold climates. Neither high-protein nor high-carbohydrate intakes can effectively do this.

Mrs. Hunt's recent dietary history, surprisingly enough, appeared to represent a food intake adequate in calories and protein, and about average in fat content. Around 20 per cent of her calories came from fat, about 60 per cent from carbohydrate, and 20 per cent from protein, a balance of nutrients that one might expect would meet her requirements.

She revealed one clue of possible significance, however. She said that her eating habits hardly ever varied. She was one of those methodical housewives who prepared weekly menus from a file of meal plans that she had developed through the years. In other words, the meals she would serve in a given week in August might be very much like those she would serve in January when the temperature was almost fifty degrees colder.

When I questioned her on this point she said, "Why, yes! We know what we like, and the number of possibilities don't afford much variation."

I told her that seasonal climatic changes ordinarily require compensatory dietary changes, very cold (or hot) weather affecting one's energy requirements.

She responded to this with what struck me as perverse reasoning: "I'm sure my depression and despondency hasn't anything at all to do with my diet or my metabolism, for I'm eating the very same things that I ate last year, and last year I felt very good—cheerful and happy, all through the holidays."

But December the previous year had been one of the warmest in the records of the weather bureau. On Christmas day, for example, the temperature rose to about eighty-five. This was one of the first things I had recalled when her husband had told me his wife hadn't had the "holiday blues" last year.

I experienced a most difficult time with Mrs. Hunt. She had a romantic, poetic, and spiritual orientation toward life, and it was almost beyond her to accept even the possibility that the loss of body heat could have any bearing on what she called her "innermost self."

She appeared almost aghast when I told her that the first thing she must do to relieve her depression would be to increase proportionally the fat content of her diet and reduce the carbohydrates.

She asked, "Are you seriously suggesting that my spiritual melancholy during this period of religious dedication results from eating toast instead of bacon for breakfast?"

I tried to explain the functional capacity of the nervous system to create energy at an optimum rate, and the body's need for adequate and proper fuel.

After considerable discussion, she tentatively accepted some dietary instructions: "Well, I really don't know—but I'll look them over."

Sometime later I had lunch with her husband, and he casually remarked, "What you said to Janet explains a lot of things."

He then told me he had known for some time that his wife always seemed "more cheerful" during the summer. He'd often wondered why Janet "loved the desert" in the winter and always wanted to go to Palm Springs for the holidays instead of sharing Christmas at home with friends and family.

He added, "It doesn't seem possible that this is all there is to it, but I also can't get over the fact that five days after she changed her diet she began calling her friends and going to social events again. She hadn't done this since before Thanksgiving."

Our blood tests had led us to classify Janet Hunt as what we called a "fast oxidizer," one who burns sugar unusually fast, with the consequent increase in the rate at which she uses up acetate. Normally this type of person suffers considerably during cold weather, unless he severely reduces his carbohydrate intake and increases his use of fatty foods such as bacon, roast pork, roast lamb, beef short ribs, and other similar foods of animal origin.

Interestingly enough, we had found that this fast-oxidizing type also reacts in a similar manner during very hot weather. One would not expect this to be true on the basis of what is known about the heat production and control mechanisms of the body, and I can only tentatively explain this unusual reaction to very hot weather on the general grounds of stress—perhaps the body must work hard to keep cool.

In view of these considerations, I was interested in following Janet Hunt's psychological progress during the coming summer. While I was relatively sure that she would fare much better emotionally during warm weather than cold, I didn't quite believe her husband's observation that she was *always* "more cheerful" during the warmer months of the year.

Consequently I scheduled brief monthly interviews with her into the summer, waiting to observe how she would react to real heat, say, ninety-five degrees or more for periods of one or two weeks.

A cool June went by, followed by a cooler July. It warmed up only slightly above normal in August, daytime highs resting in the mid-eighties. And sure enough, Mrs. Hunt was indeed cheerful and active on her new diet.

I had just about lost interest in trying to obtain information about her psychological reaction to heat as September rolled around, until one morning I glanced at the porch thermometer and saw the column of mercury standing at ninety-five degrees—and this was at seven thirty in the morning!

By two in the afternoon it was one hundred and thirteen degrees—the hottest anybody had ever dreamed or heard of around Pasadena. The next five days were all well over a hundred, followed by a week or so of temperatures in the mid-nineties.

I waited to hear from the Hunts. I was relatively certain that Janet would be suffering from another spell of what her husband had called the "holiday blues"—only this time he would have to find a different psychological reason, since these were the first weeks in September, not the Christmas holidays.

About a week went by with no word from Professor Hunt or from his wife. My curiosity finally impelled me to phone him and ask how everything was going.

"Pretty good," he said. "Janet looks like she's working out some of her old psychological problems again." He said his wife had been quite depressed lately, with a morbid interest in the past, "dwelling on what might have been."

I felt guilty for not having kept in closer touch. "Why didn't you call me about this?"

After a pause he said, "Well, for one thing, she isn't *freezing*, is she?"

In addition to those psychochemical responses that result from extremes in temperature, other climatic factors may also influence adversely the production of energy in the central nervous system. Best known among these are weather fronts—storms—and what may be called the "electrical" character of the atmosphere, such as the ionization.

Unfortunately, this whole subject of the effect of weather on the human organism is most complex and little understood. However, for our present purposes we need only to recognize one basic rule: Any sharp shift in the weather tends to further disturb one's metabolism in the direction toward which it normally tends.

We had found that Mrs. Hunt was a very fast oxidizer, one who broke down sugar in the tissues unusually rapidly, with a resultant depletion of her stores of the energy-rich intermediate acetate. This means, for example, that a cold storm front bringing rain would further increase the rate at which she burned sugar and further increase her needs for acetate. Now, unless she was aware of this and cut down her carbohydrate intake and increased her fat intake, she would find herself nervous, irritable, anxious, and depressed.

On the other hand, if Mrs. Hunt had been what we call a "slow oxidizer," her problems would have been reversed. Slow oxidizers burn carbohydrates inefficiently, rather than too fast, and a diet that contains too much fat and protein causes trouble; for, unless sugar is being broken down normally, neither fat nor protein can be turned into energy. A cold storm front bringing rain seems to further increase the need for the breakdown of sugar. Unless a slow oxidizer knows this and cuts down on the fat and protein intake, while increasing the carbohydrate intake, the adverse psychological results that follow may be similar to those indicated above.

What we have called "slow" and "fast" oxidizers are "psychochemical types"—people who do not react normally to an average or ordinary diet. We will discuss psychochemical types in detail later, and show how you can determine whether you fall into one of these categories. It is important to know your own psychochemical type in order to know what psychological reactions to *expect* from such abnormal weather conditions as heat, cold, and storms, as well as to know what to do to help yourself.

This kind of information would have saved both Gerald and Janet Hunt a great deal of misery, which directly resulted from misunderstanding the nature and cause of Mrs. Hunt's depressions. These melancholy periods did not originate in her unconscious mind, and they had no psychological significance for either her past or her present life.

In addition to the weather, there are other rather common environmental causes of abnormal mental and emotional responses that go almost entirely unrecognized.

I recall the unusual case of John Marks, a thirty-five-year-old man who had recently won a big promotion to West Coast manager of a large national corporation. An appropriate increase in salary led to the purchase of a new home in one of the exclusive residential areas. The house was on spacious, landscaped grounds, requiring the weekly services of a professional gardener.

Mr. Marks assumed his new position with enthusiasm and performed his duties with ease and considerable success. Everything seemed to be fine—for a while.

Then he began to come home exhausted, almost to the point of nausea. But soon he recovered, and he forgot about it.

A couple of weeks later he arrived home from work feeling normally tired, but good. It was a Friday; his wife was attending a club meeting. It was a warm night in June, and after dinner, while sitting out in the patio looking over the spacious gardens, he suddenly felt unaccountably excited. His thoughts began racing through unrelated fantasies, and soon he felt overcome with a nameless fear.

My God, he said to himself, *something's happening—something's going to happen. . . .* He began to sweat and to take deep breaths. He felt scared, really scared. He was miserable—hot, sweating, wild, and panicky. He wiped the sweat from his forehead.

Looking at the sweat, the thought of a steam bath occurred to him. His bathroom contained a large stall shower that had a tile bench in it. He got into the shower, turned the spray on hot, and directed it against the opposite wall. He sat on the tile bench, and was soon dripping wet with sweat in the cloud of steam generated by the hot shower playing against the tile.

Gradually he felt himself relaxing—"coming out of it," he said. The wild, racing thoughts began to give way to more normal mental patterns, then suddenly he seemed to just "snap back" to being himself.

He looked around in surprise, wondering what had happened, wondering why he was in the shower. And he began to worry. *Am I cracking up?* he asked himself.

He took a sedative and went to bed, and the next morning felt almost normal, but a little jittery. He had to go out of town on business for several days, and by the time he returned home he felt good and had just about forgotten the whole incident.

But not quite, for every once in a while a small inner voice would say: *If it happened once, it can happen again.*

The days slipped by, however, and the increasing responsibilities of his new position soon obscured the feared event of the past.

It was another Friday evening, his wife's club night, and he was out walking in the garden. Suddenly the whole scene began again—the initial surge of excitement, the racing mental fantasies, followed by engulfing fear. And all of this was accompanied by the same intense physical discomfort and heavy perspiration as before.

Once more he saved himself in a cloud of steam, sitting dripping with sweat on the tile bench in the shower.

Now he was sure something was really wrong. The next day he called his physician, told him what had happened, and asked for the most complete medical examination it was possible to obtain. To his surprise, as well as to his relief, his doctor told him that such an examination would require a five-day stay in the hospital, beginning the following Monday.

Mr. Marks said that the extensive tests covered every possible physical explanation for the attacks, but since they all turned out to be normal, his doctor told him that he ought to see a psychiatrist to try to find the cause of this thing.

Consequently he began a series of once-weekly psychiatric interviews, and although he had several more attacks during the summer, they became less and less frequent during the fall, and by the end of the year appeared to stop altogether. He then discontinued his conferences with the psychiatrist.

I asked him what had developed during these psychiatric interviews, and he told me that the psychiatrist had once asked him, "Has it ever occurred to you that you really don't *want* to succeed?" Although he didn't come right out and say so, Mr. Marks got the impression that the psychiatrist believed that his attacks were the expression of an unconscious desire to fail in his new position, a notion he dismissed as ludicrous.

During the winter months there was no trouble of any kind; in fact, Mr. Marks worked so well that he was given a new contract with another substantial increase in salary. The past, while presenting a mystery, seemed over and gone.

That is, until one warm, spring evening when Mr. Marks felt that peculiar feeling of excitement begin again. This attack ultimately led to his volunteering to become one of our research patients. He said that he had always believed that there must be some physical reason for his attacks, principally because they could be relieved so dramatically by something as simple as a sweat bath.

In our initial interview he made one remark that finally led to the discovery of the cause of his acute mental and emotional episodes.

He said, "I know this will sound crazy, but what puzzles me is that these spells only happen in the evening and only on Friday!" He was absolutely sure of these points.

Since Friday was also the night his wife went out to a club meeting, his psychiatrist had suggested a connection between the wild feelings of panic and a long-repressed fear of being abandoned by his mother, now transferred to his wife.

I asked him to tell me if there was anything else that happened only on Friday evenings. For example, did he possibly drink something exotic once in a while to relax after a hard week, something that he might be allergic to? He said he didn't drink, and didn't eat anything unusual.

The only thing he could think of was that Friday usually marked the end of a tough week—but, he protested, "I'm not beat, not worn out, when Friday rolls around. In fact, I often go to the office again Saturday morning, just to think things over when the phones aren't ringing and nobody is waiting to see me."

I was about to give up this line of inquiry and assign the Friday connection to rare coincidence when he said he had just thought of something "silly." I asked him what it was.

"The gardener comes on Friday," he said, a little sheepishly.

I learned that the gardener did indeed come Fridays, and that he sometimes brought a tank sprayer, with which he sprayed all of the shrubs with a pesticide (parathion) to control insects.

This particular chemical happens to be one of the strongest insecticides in use, and one that is perhaps among the most toxic to humans. The effects that result from inhalation include nausea, weakness, sweating, breathing failure, and mental disturbances. Mr. Marks had experienced all of these symptoms. Yet when I suggested to him that this was undoubtedly the cause of his mysterious attacks, he asked, "How could such a chemical affect my mind?"

I told him that it affected the nervous system by disrupting the normal energy-producing activity of the cells and thus interfering with the transmission of nerve impulses.

Although parathion and other strong insecticides (such as chlordane and malathion) are known to produce acute reactions in the central nervous system, there are other poisons in common use in the home that may also unexpectedly induce psychochemical responses.

I recall Mrs. R., a middle-aged woman whom we studied as a case of severe depression accompanied by hallucinations. At times she said she could actually see and touch her parents, who had died many years ago.

What was most unusual about Mrs. R. was that she not only had no history of previous mental or emotional trouble, but that these symptoms appeared so suddenly. It seemed to me that this last consideration ought to be looked into, for there must have been some precipitating circumstance to bring on her severe symptoms so quickly.

I learned that just before she became ill her husband had suffered a stroke requiring intensive twenty-four-hour nursing care.

They hired three nurses, who each worked an eight-hour shift, and Mrs. R. moved into her husband's bedroom to "see that everything went all right."

One might suspect that the strain this ordeal placed on Mrs. R. was great enough to exhaust her both physically and emotionally, resulting in her "nervous breakdown."

But she said that this was not so. She missed neither sleeping nor eating, and although she was worried about her husband, she said that this was nothing new, for she had been through other troubles before and she "always worried about him."

It was only a few days after we had accepted Mrs. R. as a patient that she telephoned and said treatment would have to wait, for they were leaving town for a month, going to their summer home at Lake Arrowhead. She thought the change would be good for her, and the doctor wanted her husband to go and forget all about his business affairs for a while. She promised to call me when they returned, which she did.

I was a bit surprised when she told me she was feeling fine. "The vacation did wonders for me," she said, and her tone of voice confirmed it.

One rarely sees a patient appear to recover from a severe mental and emotional disturbance in such a short period of time under almost any circumstances—much less without treatment. When a person's metabolic machinery is disturbed, it takes some definite remedial action to bring it back to normal.

However, I was again surprised when she telephoned for an appointment two weeks later, saying, "All of my troubles have come back."

I probably would never have understood why she suddenly had become ill, suddenly appeared to have recovered, and then suddenly became ill again if her husband hadn't accompanied her for her appointment.

He waited in the outer reception room, a rather small, poorly ventilated enclosure, for perhaps thirty or forty minutes. At the end of Mrs. R.'s interview I accompanied her to the reception room to speak to her husband.

As I opened the door I was engulfed by a most oppressive odor, which I recognized at once to be naphthalene, a crystalline hydrocarbon used as a moth repellent and in the making of dyes.

I said, "It's awfully close in here, isn't it? And oddly enough, it smells of moth balls."

Mr. R. put his hand in his left suit-coat pocket and with a grin produced a small handful of moth balls!

He turned out to be fanatic on the subject of moths, and actually claimed that he bought moth balls and moth crystals in hundred-pound cartons in order to protect his valuable wardrobe. He wore only four-hundred-dollar tailored suits, his wife told me, and he had dozens of them hanging in the extensive closets in his bedroom.

Mrs. R. told me that she normally lived in another wing of the house and couldn't "stand the smell of moth balls." Since her husband's illness, however, she had moved into his bedroom suite, where even the rugs, she said, were sprinkled with moth crystals.

When I suggested to them that it was a most dangerous practice to expose themselves constantly to air heavily laden with particles of naphthalene, since it was very toxic and known to be a nervous-system depressant, Mr. R. just shrugged.

He said, "It doesn't bother me one bit—and I don't even notice the smell. And besides, I have ten thousand dollars' worth of clothes in those closets, and if you think I'm going to let the moths eat them, you'd better think again!"

People vary widely in their sensitivity and in their psychological reactions to poisons such as naphthalene. While some persons are easily able to detoxify rather large intakes of such a poison, others appear equally unable to tolerate even small amounts. Mrs. R. was one of the latter, for the naphthalene-laden atmosphere in her husband's bedroom most certainly did affect her, and in fact appeared to be the sole cause of her depression and other mental symptoms.

When she moved back into her own rooms in the opposite wing of the house, she began to improve almost immediately, and within a few weeks she felt as good as she had when they returned from their month in the mountains.

These last two illustrations have presented rather extreme examples of psychochemical responses, resulting from the somewhat unusual and indiscriminate use of toxic chemicals. However, abnormal mental and emotional reactions may result from what might appear to be the "normal" use of pesticides.

I was asked by a friend to evaluate the behavior of his fourteen-year-old daughter, who had suddenly begun talking in a wild, babbling manner during a study period at school.

Our laboratory tests indicated that her oxidation rate was considerably depressed, a finding unusual in adolescents, for they generally have little trouble burning sugar.

When I told her father this, he asked us if we would run our tests on both himself and his wife, because, he said, "Everyone in the family has been acting kind of crazy. We're all irritable, jumpy, and extrasensitive to criticism, almost paranoid at times."

We found that all three—father, mother, and daughter—had similarly disturbed biochemical profiles, suggesting the possibility of a common source of difficulty.

The family had just moved into a country house, and they had found it teeming with spiders. The father had repeatedly sprayed every inch of the place—the ceilings, closets, under all of the beds, with a well-known insect killer.

When I told him about the psychological hazards of using such poisonous chemicals around living areas, he said that such a connection had never occurred to him. He also said, "Now that you mention it, I guess our troubles *did* begin after we moved out here. Nothing like this ever happened when we were in the apartment in town."

I suggested that they take a short vacation, leaving the house to ventilate for a week or so, and under any circumstances not to move back until all traces of the odor of the pesticide were gone.

A couple of months later I received a thank-you note saying they were "themselves" again, and promising to treat potentially dangerous household chemicals with far more caution in the future.

Probably the most commonly encountered toxic source of psychochemical trouble is also the one least likely to be regarded as dangerous.

I first became aware of this problem many years ago, in fact quite soon after I began studying some of the relationships between body chemistry and behavior.

I received an urgent telephone call one morning from one of our most valued patients. We had studied Mary B. as a case of spontaneous (endogenous) depression. She was twenty-nine, apparently in good health, and had gradually found herself becoming more and more depressed "for no reason at all."

She was happily married and the mother of two children, a boy seven and a girl nine. She responded rapidly to the nutritional therapy we were using at the time. At the end of a brief period of three months she described herself as "*more* than recovered, since I feel better now than I can ever remember having felt."

This is why I referred to her as one of our most valued patients. When we help someone we are not only encouraged and rewarded by a successful response, but also we learn more about helping someone else.

Consequently the urgent telephone call from Mary B. telling me that she had suddenly relapsed into despair and depression came as a real shock. How could she have been happy and well only a few days ago and very disturbed today if we had indeed restored her to something resembling biochemical health?

I asked her to come to the lab so that we could make some tests to see whether we could find anything we might consider abnormal. The results looked very much like those we had obtained when we first began working with her. She was burning sugar very fast again, while only two weeks ago she had been normal.

I asked her to tell me everything that had happened just before she began to feel depressed. Her answer was: "Nothing *bad* happened at all. In fact, something *good* happened. My husband got a few days off and decided to do some things around the house that I have wanted him to do for years."

It turned out that he had painted the bedroom, the living room, the kitchen, and the bathroom. It was winter, the weather was cold and damp, and they kept the windows closed and stayed in that little house breathing heavy paint fumes for almost a week.

This was my first encounter with someone who became temporarily emotionally ill by breathing the fumes of drying paint. I have since that time witnessed a great range of psychochemical responses that resulted when sensitive people were exposed to drying paint fumes. The most common reactions are irritability and excitement, followed by depression, nausea, and loss of appetite (anorexia).

One should expect to find that such common household items as ammonia, pesticides, and paints can cause psychochemical responses, since they interfere with cellular enzymes and thus directly disturb the energy-producing abilities of the tissues. There are, however, many nonpoisonous substances in our environment that can also cause mental and emotional trouble.

Recently a writer friend gave his wife permission to redecorate his study. He had just received an advance of $5,000 on a novel. His work was progressing very well, his confidence was high, and the receipt of the check resulted in a surge of optimism.

It didn't last long. Soon after his workroom had been done over (in a kind of tropical motif with heavy, woven grass floor mats and brightly colored rattan furniture), he found himself in a mental slump. The normal creative flow of words and ideas gradually slowed to a virtual halt. He simply couldn't think.

As the days, then the weeks, slipped by, while the pile of manuscript pages failed to grow, his mood of despondency turned to desperation.

He would sit at his desk in a blank mental fog for an hour or so, then leave the house for a long walk along the shore of the bay. Once, after being gone for several hours, he returned home feeling considerably clearer of mind, and actually wrote a couple of pages before his flow of words blocked again.

In addition to being depressed about his work, he also noted that his appetite had changed. Things that he used to enjoy, such as a mid-morning cup of hot tea, now tasted as if it had been brewed from old straw or hay. Also he found himself suddenly unable to remain in a room where someone was smoking. Cigarettes were bad enough, but cigar smoke was suffocating.

One morning he felt so bad that he was afraid of what he might do in desperation. Sitting at his desk, he suddenly felt that he couldn't breathe. He grabbed his jacket and left for a long walk along the tidelands. As he walked, he gradually began to breathe more easily, and at the same time the curtain of mental depression began to lift.

He returned home feeling much better, and when he opened the door to his study he was struck by the heavy oppressive air in the room. The place smelled like a hayloft on a hot August afternoon. At that moment he had a flash of insight. "It's those damned grass mats!" he yelled.

In a fury he carried all of the rattan furniture into the garage, dragging the heavy woven-grass mats after it. He flung open all the windows and took deep breaths of the cool sea air rushing in from the bay, and then he sat down, tired and dripping sweat, but vastly relieved mentally.

His flash of insight turned out to be correct. It *was* the mats. He was allergic to them, and while the tiny particles that arose from them to fill the air were not literally poisonous, they might just as well have been as far as he was concerned.

To most of us, the mention of "allergy" makes us think of sneezing, red runny noses, and tear-stained eyes. These are, of course, associated with hay fever, one of the most common kinds of allergic reactions.

There are many other kinds of hypersensitivities to foreign substances (principally proteins), however, that may not be recognized as allergies. For example, allergic reactions may affect the heart, stomach, bowels, skin, nervous system—in fact, they may disrupt practically every major physiological system in the body.

The role of allergens (substances causing allergic reactions) as causes of psychochemical responses is an almost unexplored area of study. Part of the reason is, of course, neglect, largely owing to the prevalent mentalistic orientation of both psychiatry and clinical psychology.

Another reason why few scientists have concerned themselves with the possibility that some abnormal mental and emotional reactions are allergenic in origin is that it is most difficult to establish definite cause-effect relationships between an offending substance and the supposed allergic reaction.

The number of possible allergens—such as dusts of various kinds, dog hair, horse hair, cat hair, textiles, synthetic fibers, pollens from a myriad of plants and trees, as well as literally hundreds of food items—all make the study of allergic reactions difficult and exhausting. Often it is easier for the patient to find the offending allergen, as the novelist did in the preceding case history, than it might be for a specialist. Through the years I have had many research patients who have been able to observe their own abnormal psychological reactions under certain conditions, leading them to believe that their mental and emotional upsets have had some obscure physical causes.

We interviewed an artist who said that whenever he visited the mountains for any length of time he would be overcome with intense fear, at times approaching panic. When this happened he said he felt that he was going to lose control of himself and maybe physically assault someone. During such an attack he found it hard to breathe. He said that he couldn't get enough air to satisfy him. Because of this last symptom he thought that perhaps the "thin mountain air" affected his brain and caused the fears and panic.

I had to admit that such a thing was possible; however, it was most unlikely, since the altitude at which he experienced his attacks was only 5,000 feet, hardly high enough to cause noticeable difficulty in breathing.

Since respiratory depression (difficulty in breathing) is one of the most common kinds of allergic reactions, I asked him whether he had any allergies.

Indeed he had, he said, "roses and Christmas trees—both make me feel like I'm going to catch cold." His eyes watered, and he sneezed and coughed if he remained for long in a room where there were roses or a Christmas tree.

This information provided a definite clue that possibly pointed to the source of his "mountain panic."

"Christmas tree" might mean Douglas fir (or some other evergreen), and these trees covered the slopes of the resort areas where he felt strangely afraid and panicky.

When I suggested to him the possibility that his fears in the mountains might be a psychochemical response to the particles in the air which came from the pine trees, he seemed definitely relieved.

"You know," he said, "I've really been worried sometimes. I've tried to tell myself that my bad mental reactions were due to the thin mountain air, but I knew this couldn't be the whole story. Just before I came to see you I visited an artist friend and had one of the most miserable times of my life."

It seems that his artist friend lived in the beautiful pine forest outside of Cambria. But this forest is not in the mountains. His friend's house was on a low cliff overlooking the ocean—but it was surrounded by a lush stand of pine trees.

Earlier it was stated that any interference with the nutritional supply lines or with the energy-producing systems of the brain results in impaired functioning and in those abnormal mental and emotional reactions that are psychochemical responses. Since infectious illness, such as influenza or even the common cold, both disrupts one's nutrition (mainly owing to loss of appetite) and reduces the ability of the tissues to produce energy, one should not be surprised to find that virtually all such sickness is accompanied by adverse mental and emotional reactions.

Although this observation appears to me to be clear and simple, I keep rediscovering that there are many people who just don't think in such obvious terms.

Some time ago we employed a very bright young man as a laboratory assistant. Allan was a graduate student in psychology, and he had a talent for seeing through things, for spotting connections that others missed.

Since Allan was mentally quick and full of fresh ways of looking at things, I was always interested in what he might say. One day he casually told me that he could predict at least two days in advance when he was going to catch cold—that is, two days before there were any cold symptoms at all, when nose, eyes, and throat were still absolutely normal. "You know," he said, "to someone like you, this might sound fishy. But here it is, for what you want to make of it."

He told me that while he usually was a very cheerful person, there were times when he became "quite sad for no reason at all." For example, he generally drove his car with the radio playing. He could spot the beginning of one of these periods of sadness when tears welled up in his eyes when certain songs were played, songs that touched a tender point in his past. Normally these same songs didn't affect him at all. But when this happened, he would come down with a cold in about two days. I asked him if sadness was the only psychological change that preceded a cold.

"No, not at all," he said, "but it is the *clearest.* I mean I almost can't miss on this clue. But in addition, I may be very apprehensive, anxious, or even afraid. And when there is absolutely no reason for me to feel this way, I can almost count on coming down with a cold in a couple of days."

When I asked him how he accounted for the apparent connection between feeling sad and catching cold, he said simply, "The cold is obviously psychosomatic. My thoughts and feelings have the ability to make me *physically* ill."

I didn't laugh at this, for I liked him too well to hurt his feelings. But to me his depression and anxiety were psychochemical responses, reflecting disturbed body processes. Allan already "had" the cold when he felt sad, although he didn't know it until he sneezed a few times.

So I asked him if he'd like to make a little wager. I would bet that I not only could "predict" when he was going to have a cold, but I also could at the same time tell him when he felt sad, apprehensive, or fearful.

This time *he* laughed. But I wasn't joking.

We agreed to a little experiment. He was to come to the lab without breakfast on random days of his own choice and let us have a blood sample. On the basis of our tests I would try to tell him whether he felt emotionally normal with no cold in sight, or sad and depressed with a cold coming on.

Allan thought this was going to be great fun. What he failed to remember when we made our wager was that he had very few colds, maybe only one or two a winter.

The first week he showed up twice for pre-breakfast blood tests. Both times I told him the tests looked good. No sadness. No cold.

He kept up the two tests a week for more than a month, and since I kept telling him everything looked normal, he adopted a new tack. He quit coming for tests. I figured he was now going to wait until he was in a "sad period" and then try to call my bluff.

A couple of months went by—it was now almost spring—before Allan showed up before breakfast for another test. I again assured him that he was feeling good and wasn't going to catch cold.

He hadn't been able to fool us on one end of the wager, at any rate. After every test we told him that he wasn't on the verge of a cold, and he hadn't caught cold. What I wanted, however, was to win the whole game by spotting a "period of sadness," and then telling him that he was going to also catch cold. But it began to look as if Allan wasn't going to have a cold this year, after all, for winter was now gone.

He surprised me one warm morning in late spring, for he showed up for what he said was his "last try. I guess our bet is about a stand-off," he said. "The cold season is about over."

The lab report showed that Allan's oxidation rate had shifted sharply; the rate at which his tissues were burning sugar was now way below normal. We had never received a report of this kind on him before. And through the years we had observed many patients with colds, or "coming down" with colds, whose oxidation rates had shifted in this same manner.

So I called Allan, and asked him to come to my office.

"Well?" he asked.

"You'd better plan to take at least three days off," I said, "and be sure to stay warm and drink plenty of liquids."

He just looked at me for a few seconds, and then he said, "If I didn't feel so damned low, I'd laugh instead of cry."

The case histories we have been considering illustrate some of the kinds of psychochemical responses that result either from inadequate nutrition or from the inability of the cells to create energy normally, owing to toxic, allergic, or infectious interference.

While it is true that proper nutrition and freedom from chemical interference with the operation of the nervous system are essential to normal mental and emotional health, they alone do not guarantee it.

Some years ago we helped a young woman patient recover from a severe depression and "nervous breakdown" (she called it) that occurred following the birth of her first child. She had responded quickly and fully to the nutritional treatment she received, and in our last interview asked me, "Is there anything you can do for my husband?"

She told a story that I suppose is familiar to everyone. Her husband wasn't physically or mentally ill, she said, but "he's sort of aimless, like he didn't have a rudder. He's always changing direction, and he just can't stay onto anything very long."

She then described a half-dozen different "enthusiasms" he had taken up during the past few years, only to drop them, one after the other, just as easily as he had taken them up.

For example, for a period of about six months he was going to become a stockbroker. This gave way to an interest in selling books, since the stock market wasn't "mentally challenging." Suddenly the idea of wealth through uranium captured his attention, and he spent a half-dozen weekends in hot, rough desert country with a Geiger counter, trying to strike it rich by finding a uranium deposit. He then started negotiations for a doughnut shop franchise, saying, "People always have to eat, you know." This fell through because he couldn't raise enough capital to get started.

She listed several other temporary enthusiasms of his, concluding with the remark, "Well, I guess you get the idea by now, don't you?"

I had very little interest in the case of her husband, principally because I could think of many possible causes for his behavior. Some of these, such as inherited predispositions, would virtually eliminate the possibility of our helping him.

While I agreed to interview and test him from a general biochemical point of view, at the same time I tried to convey to her some idea of how complicated and how little understood was the whole subject of motivation and achievement.

Her husband, Jack W., turned out to be a very pleasant, likable, and seemingly intelligent young man. He was twenty-four and had completed three years toward an engineering degree. In view of his wife's comments about his lack of purpose, I didn't ask him why he hadn't finished the last year of college, as I would have liked to. But it made me wonder, for he would never have stuck it out for three years if he had been as "rudderless" then as his wife now described him as being.

Our tests and interview appeared to reveal a normally healthy young man with a good appetite and fairly sound eating habits. He said a recent medical examination had found him to be in excellent health. I asked him if there had been some special reason why he had gone for a medical checkup; and he told me that it wasn't because of illness, but that he felt he ought to have more energy. Sometimes he said he felt completely exhausted when he hadn't done anything at all.

"If I'm in excellent health, like the doctor says," he asked, "why can't I seem to wake up in the morning? I've lost more jobs by being late to work. And after lunch I can hardly keep my eyes open."

I told him that the ease with which a person could wake up and get out of bed depended directly on how long he had been asleep and how tired he had been when he had gone to bed.

He missed my point entirely.

"Don't worry," he said, "I get plenty of sleep. My problem is that I can't wake up when the alarm goes off."

When I pressed the issue he revealed that by "plenty of sleep" he meant five or six hours, from 12:30 or 1:00 A.M. to 6:00 or 6:30 A.M.

Since I doubted that this was sufficient sleep for him, I decided to give Jack a little scientific sales pitch on the importance of this passive activity.

I began by admitting that while there were many theories, but very little real knowledge, about the nature of sleep, one thing was absolutely certain: The nervous system cannot function optimally when the body is deprived of sleep. At least one reason for this is that during the wakeful hours the cells of the tissues become "tired" because of complex biochemical changes connected with the work the cells perform when one is awake.

The cells may be restored during sleep to their normal ability to function, however, if the individual is adequately nourished so that the nutritional biochemicals necessary to repair tired cells are fully available.

Consequently, if one awakens refreshed and eager to get going, he does so only because his nutrition is good and he has had enough sleep to put his nervous system back in good working order.

On the other hand, if a person can hardly drag himself out of bed, and at the moment would give a thousand dollars if he could just go back to sleep, you can be certain that this person's body and brain have not been restored sufficiently through nutrition and rest to be able to function normally.

There was a brief interval of silence after I finished my little lecture; then Jack said, "There is this fellow who lives next door —healthy, strong, always up and at 'em. And you know what? He has two full-time jobs! From seven to four as a clerk in an auto parts store, and from four thirty to twelve thirty as a waiter in an Italian restaurant!"

I ignored this comment completely, for I had heard this kind of story too many times. Instead, I asked Jack if he could swim.

"Sure, I like to swim," he replied.

I asked him how far he could swim, how many laps in a pool, or yards or even miles in the ocean.

"One or two lengths of the pool at the Y is more than enough for me," he said.

"Well," I told him, "I know a fellow who swims *fifty* lengths of the Y pool, several times a week."

In almost any factor of human behavior, obviously there is a wide range of differences between people who, on the surface, appear to be constructed along the same lines. There are some who can easily swim fifty pool-lengths, some who can't swim at all, while the vast majority of us just paddle along modestly. Most of us simply cannot do two full-time jobs a day without collapse. As for sleep, few of us can restore body and brain in only five or six hours after working even one full-time job.

A very likely cause of both Jack's difficulty in waking up in the morning and his unusual fatigue during the day was that he was not giving his body and brain the rest they needed in order to repair themselves. I also reminded him that there was no medical or scientific authority who could tell him how much sleep *he* needed to function, physically as well as mentally, at his full capacity.

The only one who is in a position to provide this information for a person is himself. He might do this by gradually increasing his nightly sleep quota until that morning arrives when he awakens refreshed, alert, and eager to meet the challenges of the day ahead.

Since I had seen small miracles happen in the lives of a number of people who tried this approach, I told Jack that he really ought to find out for himself whether or not he was literally wasting his life away, limping along physically and mentally at a much lower level of awareness and performance than he was capable of achieving.

He responded with a curious remark, one that I had heard far too many times: "I'm sleeping one-fourth of my life away, and now you're asking me to increase this to maybe one-third or even more!"

Many people are content to drag themselves through the weary hours, day after tired day, with the dimmest level of awareness, their only goal being to stay awake so they "won't miss anything."

The irony of this way of living, of course, is that these misguided individuals are in fact missing everything. Their weary eyes and numbed brains give them only a pale impression of the vivid real world around them.

Jack politely thanked me for my time and interest, told me he would think it over, and promised to call me in a week or so.

He didn't. Almost three months later, however, I received a call from his wife, who said she was mad at me. "I hardly ever get to see my husband anymore," she said. The thought struck me that the reason he hadn't called as he had promised was that he had taken a second job just to show he could handle it, like the fellow next door.

I asked her why she thought I was responsible for her not being able to spend more time with her husband.

"He *sleeps* all the time," she replied, "and he said that you told him to!"

What had happened was this: Jack began increasing his time in bed at the rate of one-half hour each night for a week, so that at the end of the first month he was retiring around 10:30 instead of 12:30, and was getting about eight hours of sleep instead of six. He said that with this much sleep he was beginning to feel a little better, but that he was also discovering that he was a lot more tired than he had ever realized.

"Once I began to let down a little," he explained, "I also began to see that I had been sort of running on nerves for years."

Consequently he decided to increase his time in bed as much as possible to see what would happen. He reached a maximum of twelve hours' sleep a night, which he maintained for about a month, before he finally felt that he was getting all the sleep he could handle.

It was during this period, when he was sleeping from seven in the evening until seven in the morning, that his wife called me to complain about being neglected.

Soon after this, however, Jack was able to reduce his sleeping to an average of nine hours and still find it fairly easy to arise in the morning and feel good all day.

Several months later, when I asked him whether his sleep experiment had helped him, he said, "I can see now that I really didn't know anything about this at all. Like you said, it *is* a totally different world, now." Reflectively he added: "And I feel like a different person."

Whenever increased physical or mental demands are imposed upon us, both our nutritional needs and our requirements for tissue repair (sleep) also increase proportionally. Energy output must be balanced by biochemical input, accompanied by the allowance for a sufficient amount of time during which the body can restore itself to its best level of functioning.

In terms of daily living this simply means that one's nutrition and rest must completely compensate for everything that one does if one is to maintain the same level of performance from day to day.

While the number of ways that people can discover to overextend themselves is probably almost as great as the total number of people, there are some basic patterns of stress that are extremely common.

One very common but almost entirely misunderstood type of disturbed behavior carries the fearsome title "postpartum psychosis," or "postpartum blues." Quite frequently women who have just borne a child become emotionally disturbed, threatening harm to both themselves and their offspring. Current psychiatric thinking attributes such behavior to deep unconscious conflicts, possibly stemming from repressed infantile sexual drives. On the other hand, we have successfully treated postpartum mental and emotional disturbances by viewing them as psychochemical responses resulting from the depletion of the mother's nutritional biochemical reserves.

Pregnancy and childbirth present the most obvious example of increased needs for massive biochemical support. Even with the best prenatal nutrition, however, mothers often find themselves emotionally and physically exhausted after childbirth. The prenatal special diet which has been followed to ensure the birth of a healthy normal baby is now abandoned–with no thought given to the newly created requirements of the postpartum mother, who should be given intensive nutritional replacement therapy to restore her tissues to normal (see Chapter V for suggested diet and nutritional supplements).

Perhaps the most frequently encountered everyday cause of abnormal mental and emotional reactions owing to stress is "overcommitment," the attempt to carry out a daily life plan that is clearly beyond one's mental, emotional, and physical resources.

This particular kind of overcommitment is the sick life pattern of large cities, where one's transportation to and from work, the job itself, plus those things to do at home, far exceed one's ability to daily absorb stress and recover fully within a twenty-four-hour period.

People so overcommitted find themselves a little more tired each morning as the week unfolds; they thank God for Friday. But each succeeding Monday morning they start out again. They may not be aware of it at the time, but they are a little less able to maintain the pace at the same level of performance as the weeks and months go by. It generally takes a few years before this kind of gradual biochemical erosion results in real physical and psychological trouble, but such an outcome is inevitable.

A very good friend called and asked me if I would do him a favor. He said he knew one of the most talented, most intelligent, and most gifted young women in Hollywood, Doris James, who was in desperate need of help. "She isn't going to make it, the way it looks right now," he said.

He also told me that she had been to "all the doctors" and had been going to a psychiatrist for three years, and yet she was becoming more and more upset.

I agreed to look into the case.

Mrs. James arrived for her initial interview on a cold, rainy Saturday morning. She was a frail wisp of a girl who that morning looked like a wet kitten. I met her in the waiting room, where she acknowledged my hello with a nod, without even looking at me.

I led the way to my office. She sat down, took off her gloves, and began to cry. Finally exhausted, and out of tears, she apologized and began to talk.

What I heard was an almost endless list of "impossibles." Her position as a writer, although she was among the highest-paid writers in the country, was "impossible." Her husband, a successful lawyer, was also "impossible," even though she said she admired and respected him. "He's kind, gentle, understanding, and helpful." She paused, then sighed. "But he's *impossible!* I never should have married him."

Their home, which I later discovered was a small mansion in Encino, was "just simply impossible."

As the list of things she found intolerable grew, it became clear to me that the real truth was that perhaps none of these things was impossible.

As a rule, when every aspect of one's life situation seems to be at fault, the most likely reason is to be found within the person himself.

When Mrs. James finally finished her long list of complaints, I asked, "Has it occurred to you that you haven't made a single reference to *yourself* in all that you've told me?"

Our subsequent discussion revealed what was really wrong in the life of Doris James. She had previously mentioned that her car, "on top of everything else," was "impossible." I asked her what she meant.

"Well," she said, "I have this *prestige* car"—she emphasized the word—"that has a stick shift and is awfully tiring for me to drive in stop-and-go traffic. I'm simply worn out by the time I get to the studio in the morning."

When I asked her why she didn't drive a car with an automatic transmisssion, she gave me a funny look and asked, "Do you mean something like a *Chevy?*" To Doris James such an idea was clearly preposterous.

Her own self-image could be reflected only by something exotic, exclusive, and expensive–like the ten-thousand-dollar foreign sports car with the stick shift, even though it, too, was "impossible."

I soon discovered that the Doris James who appeared to be a frail wisp of a young lady was in fact only a façade that hid a driving, status-craving ego. She simply *had* to have the best husband, the best home, the best friends ("I know most of the *right* people in town"), the best job, the best clothes, the best car–everything.

There appeared to be no end to the list of things she coveted and was determined to get by her own efforts. She was well on her way to fulfilling most of her desires when she began to cave in emotionally. And after exhausting herself in their pursuit, she now found herself confronted by impossibilities wherever she looked.

This unusually bright young woman had consulted a psychiatrist for three years trying to find out "why" everything that had formerly seemed so desirable, so *necessary,* now turned out to be "impossible."

I told her that she had been looking for an answer in the wrong place, for there wasn't any psychological reason for her reactions. As a matter of fact, everything is impossible to *anyone* who lacks the mental and emotional strength to make normal responses. It takes strength to enjoy anything–and the higher the capacity for energy output of the nervous system, the greater is the ability to respond with interest, appreciation, and enjoyment to the good things around us.

When I outlined our rehabilitation program for her, emphasizing the absolute necessity of sharply curtailing the range of her frenetic activities, while increasing her tissue repair time to a minimum of ten hours' sleep a night, she said, "But I thought–at least the analysts say–that sleep is a form of escape!"

Mrs. James successfully followed the program we outlined for her, which consisted of an intensive nutritional program, together with a realistic balance between her average daily energy output and her allowance for tissue rebuilding in sleep.

She received a totally unexpected reward for facing up to the biochemical realities of her life. In addition to regaining her mental and emotional balance, she discovered that her creativity as a writer appeared to improve. She cited what I thought was reasonably objective evidence for this belief, for within the year she completed a very successful book, her first. When I asked her why she had never tried a book-length manuscript before, she replied, "I never thought I could. Every time I considered the idea in the past the task simply appeared too big. I just couldn't face it."

Probably most—if not all—of the psychochemical responses illustrated in this chapter could have been controlled by the individuals involved had they been sufficiently informed concerning some of the basic facts about how the mind and the body function.

Any type of unusual emotional reaction raises a question about the ability of the central nervous system to create energy normally. If a person is not physically ill—and none of the individuals we have been talking about were—then one must look for the causes of unusual mental and emotional reactions in the four general areas we have been discussing: 1) inadequate nutrition; 2) chemical interference with the ability of tissues to function normally, owing to drugs, poisons, allergies, or infections; 3) stress—including pregnancy and childbirth—the expenditure of mental or physical effort beyond one's biochemical limits; and 4) failure to repair tissues because of lack of sufficient sleep which is necessary to restore the cells' normal ability to create energy.

Psychochemical behavior ranges from simple moodiness to extreme abnormality. In between lie a large number of conditions, such as lack of confidence, lack of ambition, vague fears, shyness, apathy, sadness, anger, irritability, and feelings of distrust and suspicion that puzzle and disturb the person who experiences them because he can neither understand nor control them.

The possible causes of such psychochemical responses are many. Since individuals can be sorted into basic psychochemical types, however, it is possible to learn one's own psychochemical type, and then learn to recognize and to control one's own reactions.

The achievement of this kind of understanding can literally change one's life for the better. The only way to eliminate unwanted thoughts, feelings, and actions in an otherwise healthy person is to eliminate the real conditions that are responsible for them. How this may be done will be discussed in the following chapters.

III Personality Strength and Nutrition

I met Bob Walsh quite by accident, at a large, noisy "meet the artist" reception held in one of the older mansions in the Los Angeles Wilshire district. Since the party was given by a socialite patron of the university, some faculty members, myself included, were reluctantly on hand.

I detached myself from the throng milling around in the great hall and discovered a pleasant library that appeared to be unoccupied. I entered and closed the door behind me on the voices of the crowd.

I selected a book, sank down in a deep chair, and soon was mentally far away. But every little while I fancied I heard something quite near. Suddenly it sneezed.

Hidden in another deep chair across the room was a thin, ascetic-looking young man, who apologized for disturbing me.

Bob was a twenty-five-year-old Ph.D. dropout. After achieving a high scholastic record as an undergraduate, he had completed a year's study toward a doctor's degree in mathematics when he was drafted.

I asked him why he hadn't gone back to the university to obtain his doctorate after getting out of the Army, and he told me that he had returned home a changed man.

"When I look back on my college years," he said, "I almost think it must have been somebody else. I was really active and ambitious. I used to go to plays and concerts, I read constantly, and yet my thoughts were never far away from math." He paused and shook his head slightly. "But I guess that's all in the past. Now I have no goals, no ambition, I hardly ever go anywhere, haven't read a book in three years, and I've simply forgotten all about math. It hardly seems possible that a *person* could change so much."

He put heavy emphasis on the word *person,* as if to convey the idea that a person ought to be something substantial, like a redwood tree that goes on being a redwood tree throughout the centuries.

My own research has provided ample evidence to the contrary. A "person" is what one thinks, feels, and does. Although one can indeed learn certain habits, they are habits only as long as one continues them. Since all behavior depends on the production of energy in the tissues, one's "personality"—what one thinks, feels, and does—changes when this energy output changes.

Bob Walsh's "intellectual" personality, his interests in the theater, concerts, literature, and mathematics, had been supported by a certain high level of brain and nervous system functioning. Obviously something had happened to lower the amount of energy his nervous system was now capable of producing.

I suggested that he might like us to run some tests on him in the hope we might possibly come up with some explanation for his personality changes.

"I appreciate your interest and all that," he said, "but I wouldn't want to waste your time. You see, my brother is a doctor, and there's nothing physically wrong with me. He says I'm 100 per cent."

I just laughed at this and told him that both he and his brother were a little naïve to believe that the art of medicine was presently advanced enough to allow such an evaluation.

At the time I met Bob Walsh our work was directed toward the study of the effects of certain vitamins on behavior, particularly those vitamins that were known to play a part in the release of energy from food.

One of the most important of these is pantothenic acid, the name deriving from the Greek, meaning "from everywhere," since this vitamin is found in virtually all foods. Pantothenic acid, a member of the vitamin-B complex, plays a key role in both of the major energy-producing cycles in the tissues.

Earlier it was pointed out that cellular energy is not derived from food directly, but rather from "intermediates," the richest of which in yielding energy is acetate. You may recall that about 80 per cent of the total energy available from glucose actually comes in the form of acetate.

This complex substance contains the B vitamin pantothenic acid, in the absence of which the acetate level of the cells decreases sharply. For example, in rats deprived of sufficient pantothenic acid, the cellular acetate level drops about 40 per cent. Strangely, very little is known about the human requirements for this vitamin. An average diet of 2,500 calories will provide about 10 milligrams of pantothenic acid, but our research suggests that this may not be sufficient to support the highest energy-producing capacity of the cells. In addition, the best sources of pantothenic acid are foods such as beef brain, heart, and liver—items not ordinarily found on the typical daily menu—so unless one knows what he is doing, it is very likely that he will select a diet that doesn't provide an average of even 10 milligrams of this important vitamin.

Our tests on Bob indicated that he apparently handled carbohydrates and fats inadequately, not oxidizing enough to provide the energy he should have been able to derive from his food. He was what we call a "suboxidizer." Although his blood tests indicated that his energy output was about 25 per cent below average, we had no direct method for determining why this was so. There were a great many possible reasons, including of course a low cellular acetate level, which as yet there is no way of measuring.

It doesn't often happen in trial-by-error clinical testing that one succeeds on the first trial. The number of ways one can be wrong is so great that one soon comes to expect frequent failure. One of the reasons, in addition to the large number of other possibilities, is that most nutritional problems involve more than just one factor. If one's diet has been inadequate over a long period of time, simply administering big doses of a single vitamin isn't likely to have much effect.

Bob Walsh was first given a bottle of tablets labeled "Calcium Pantothenate, 100 mgs.," and told to take one after breakfast each day for two weeks, while making note of any reactions, good or bad.

Bob didn't know it, but the tablets were fakes (placebos), made out of milk sugar. This beginning trial with placebos was necessary in order to eliminate the possibility that he might respond to the mere belief that the pills were helping him.

After he had taken the dummy pills for two weeks, he phoned, saying, "It's no use. I get more lift out of a couple of aspirin tablets. I'm pretty sure I don't need pantothenic acid or any other vitamin, as I first said."

I told him that I was very disappointed, for I had hoped that he would give it a longer trial. I suggested that perhaps the dose had been too small, and finally argued him into coming over and getting some different pills, this time the real thing.

Since being discharged from the army about a year before, Bob had been working in the public relations department of a large oil company. When I asked him what he did, he said, "Nothing. I just push pieces of paper from one side of my desk to the other."

Bob's paper-pushing days were numbered when he swallowed his first 100-milligram tablet of calcium pantothenate.

About ten days later, while window-shopping during his lunch hour, his eye was caught by an expensive German camera.

"It suddenly looked so beautiful, so desirable," he said, "that right then and there I decided to buy the camera and take up photography as a hobby, or maybe even as a profession."

What at first puzzled him about his sudden interest was that he had looked at that same camera dozens of times without any reaction whatsoever. In turning this point over in his mind, wondering why the unusual surge of enthusiasm, he suddenly thought, *It's the pantothenic acid!*

Electrified by this idea, and without consulting me, he decided to gradually increase the dose to see what would happen.

Believe me, it was considerable. After taking three 100-milligram tablets a day for a couple of weeks he lost all interest in the camera and photography as a hobby.

Instead, he quit his job.

He had almost $2,000 in a savings account, and he decided to "take some time off to read, think things over, and just catch up in general."

Bob continued to take 300 milligrams of calcium pantothenate a day for the next two months without my knowledge. (Although this was three times the intake I had suggested, we had tested up to ten times this amount [1,000 milligrams, or 1 gram] without observing either negative reactions or obvious additional benefits over smaller intakes.) He obtained the vitamin through his doctor brother, who thought the whole thing slightly ludicrous, however harmless. Bob later told me that his brother claimed, "Vitamins are simply high-priced placebos," apparently ignoring the biochemical operation of the human organism.

By mid-spring, five months after Bob had taken his first tablet of calcium pantothenate, he applied for readmission to his former university graduate school. Two years later he was awarded the Ph.D. degree in mathematics.

Bob Walsh subsequently investigated all of his food habits and worked to determine what diet and added vitamins and minerals would best support his mental activities at the highest level. He later told me that his intellectual performance and mathematical creativity at age twenty-seven were far better than they had ever been: he wrote his doctoral dissertation in three months, a most impressive feat. To be brighter and more creative at the age of twenty-seven than at twenty is just the reverse of what normally happens. When one knows nothing of nutrition, and eats merely from ignorance, habit, and learned prejudices, there is a steady decrease in physical—and often mental—performance as the years of youth go by.

This is a rare case, since it shows clearly how crucially important a single vitamin can be in the life of the person who needs it. The dramatic effect pantothenic acid had on Bob's personality was most likely due to a sharp increase in his cellular acetate level. Both his loss of intellectual interests and his lost ambition probably resulted from the inability of his brain cells to form acetate adequately in the absence of sufficient amounts of pantothenic acid.

I have cited this case also to illustrate two additional points.

The first is that some people—like Bob Walsh—can profitably

use far greater amounts of certain nutritional substances than an ordinary "good" diet provides.

The second, mentioned briefly before, is that your personality, what you think, feel, and do, depends to a great extent on the biochemical reactions which occur in the cells of the nervous system.

Indeed, your present pattern of life may not really reflect the "optimum you" at all, and this can result solely from nutritional needs that you know nothing about.

A friend of mine, John Gant, married an attractive, delicate, and sensitive girl. She was shy to the point of being afraid of people that she had known for years. She would go to great lengths to avoid meeting her husband's friends and business associates. This worried him considerably, and he asked me whether or not there was "anything wrong" with his wife.

Through social meetings over a rather long period of time I gradually got to know Mrs. Gant and to satisfy myself that there was "nothing wrong" with her in the psychological sense. There were no indications of abnormal mental or emotional responses in her social behavior. My friend also assured me that his wife was a happy and cheerful person in her own quiet way, and that they had a good life together.

The only trouble was that she was so afraid of everything. She refused to ride on the freeways, because she would become terrified, and at times even hysterical, in fast-moving traffic. If she purchased something that wasn't just right, she wouldn't exchange it at the store unless her husband went with her to lend moral support. She preferred to pursue her own intellectual interests at home, with as few social contacts as possible.

In reflecting on the life style of this young woman, it occurred to me that while her behavior was not frankly abnormal, she still might be exhibiting a form of psychochemical response, for her shyness and fearfulness might result from improper biochemical functioning.

I had a chance to test this idea when she mentioned in a casual conversation that it would be nice if she had more "energy," and I offered to see whether we could help her.

The psychological transformation that resulted over a period of a year would have to be seen to be believed, but you can get a general idea from noting these changes in Mrs. Gant's behavior: Instead of being afraid to ride in fast-moving traffic, she was now driving an automobile (and was given a traffic citation for speeding on a freeway); instead of being afraid of people, whether friends or strangers, she obtained a job where her principal duty was to meet the public; and instead of dreading social engagements, she complained to her husband that they didn't have enough friends to invite to dinner.

As these changes in her interests and her behavior began to occur, Mrs. Gant was frankly puzzled by them. She told me: "All my life I've thought I was an introvert. Also, that's what a psychologist told me after making some tests. But now I'm acting and thinking like an extrovert!"

In explaining the reasons behind her new "personality," I told Mrs. Gant I had seen many an alleged "introvert" turned into an "extrovert." An introvert "looks in" only because he's not creating sufficient energy in his nervous system to "look out"—to be an extrovert.

Some time later I met Mrs. Gant's mother, and she asked me, "What on earth did you ever say to my daughter? I've never seen such a change in anyone in my whole life!"

I assured her there was nothing in the world that I could say—or anybody could say—that would increase the enzyme activity in her daughter's brain cells. I told her that what we did was to provide her daughter with an optimum diet and with larger amounts of certain vitamins and minerals than she could normally obtain from her daily food intake, however good it might be.

"But," her mother protested, "my daughter doesn't need a better diet and added vitamins! Our whole family is very diet conscious and she's been raised right. Besides, I thought we got all the vitamins we need from our food. That is, we can't use any more, can we?"

Virtually no research has been done on the subject of optimum nutrition. The biochemical studies on which the present recommended (National Research Council) dietary allowances are based have all been concerned with *minimums,* not maximums. The recommended intake of a given nutrient is usually set at about 50 per cent above the bare minimum necessary for "health," which generally means nothing more than the absence of obvious nutritional disease. In this sense, it is quite true that one can achieve such a maintenance level of vitamins and minerals from an average good diet. However, a totally different question is raised when one asks whether some of us can profitably use larger amounts of vitamins and minerals than we normally get in our diet.

The Food and Nutrition Board of the National Research Council, in setting down the recommended vitamin and mineral intakes, frankly states that "the set standards are neither final nor minimal nor optimal." This statement suggests that we simply do not have enough information to allow us to say what would constitute optimum nutrition for a given individual.

Most of the studies that have been done on the effect of increased vitamin and mineral intakes on behavior have been done with rats, not humans. But even these are strongly provocative. For example, when rats were given four times their minimum need for vitamin A, the average length of life increased more than 10 per cent in the males and more than 12 per cent in the females. In addition, their "personalities" changed. They became much more "vital" and "active," indicating that they could advantageously use a much greater amount of this vitamin than they could possibly obtain from their normal "good" diet.

One of the most striking personality changes that occurs when nutrition is increased from the average toward the optimum is a change in one's goals, in one's level of aspiration. I have seen patients redirect their lives dramatically under such conditions, but inevitably the new career is dropped if the patient fails to adhere to the new nutritional program.

I have pointed out that very little research has been done on the subject of optimum nutrition as related to optimum performance in human beings. Indeed, we have seen that the recommended daily dietary allowances of the National Research Council are essentially based on a negative criterion—the absence of obvious nutritional disease.

On the other hand, I have cited case histories that illustrate a totally different way to approach the nutritional status of the individual. Rather than judging a person to be adequately nourished just as long as he doesn't show signs of rickets, pellagra, beriberi, night blindness, or some other deficiency disease, if we want to know how *well* he is nourished, we must evaluate the entire style of life he is pursuing in terms of how nearly it reflects the full energy-producing capacity of his nervous system. For it is at this level that both inferior nutrition and superior nutrition most clearly manifest themselves.

Since what is optimum nutrition for one may be grossly inadequate for another, how does one discover what are his own best levels of nutrient intake? Since in our concept of optimum nutrition the criterion of how well a person is nourished lies in his behavior, not in biochemical measurement, the only direct way for a person to determine for himself what is his best nutrition is to systematically manipulate his food and vitamin-mineral intakes and observe the results. The details of how to go about this will be given in the next chapter.

In addition to this "try and see" approach to individual optimum nutrition, there are several psychological clues that may be helpful. The following lists of contrasting attitudes, feelings, beliefs, and levels of interest and motivation are based on actually measured personality changes in research patients whose nutrition was improved from the average toward the optimum, with consequent changes in personality. Try to look at yourself as objectively as possible, and compare your own attitudes and behavior tendencies with those of both "Personality One" and "Personality Two."

Personality One (reflecting average nutrition)	Personality Two (approaching optimum nutrition)
1. Settles for security out of lack of self-confidence.	Sets high—but realistic—goals and has the confidence to take the required risks.
2. Hates to admit mistakes; the other fellow is to blame.	Admits mistakes and takes blame.
3. Mainly interested in himself and his own comfort; responds to almost everything else with indifference and apathy.	Has many interests beyond himself and generally has activities planned to look forward to.

Personality One (Cont'd)	Personality Two (Cont'd)
4. Is uncomfortable around others and avoids and tends to resent them.	Really enjoys people and actively seeks the company of others.
5. Expects the worst will happen, and dreads what the future may bring.	Looks forward to the good things the future holds in store.
6. When everything is going well, can generally find something to be pessimistic about.	In times of trouble can generally find something to be optimistic about.
7. Remembers most of the psychological scars of the past and carries them with him into the future.	Recovers from and forgets emotional blows quickly, leaving the past behind.
8. Has few friends, and can find something to criticize about everyone.	Has many friends, and accepts others for their best qualities.
9. Feels guilty and helpless about many past shortcomings.	Accepts past mistakes without feeling guilty, resolving to do better in the future.
10. Thinks life is a raw deal, and wonders why he was born at all.	Cherishes the life that has been given him, and tries to make the most of it.
11. Feels almost sure he's going to be cheated.	Expects to be treated fairly.
12. Resentful, unforgiving, and unforgetting.	Forgives quickly and easily.
13. Sensitive to real or imagined slights or criticism.	Feelings not easily hurt, tries to accept criticism objectively.
14. Emotionally flat, never really happy under the best of conditions.	Feels cheerful and happy most of the time.
15. Easily gets into arguments, feels others are "picking on him."	Tactful, tries to avoid arguments.
16. Continually puts things off, and then tends to forget them entirely.	Gets things done on time.
17. Easily forms rigid opinions without objective evidence.	Tries to be open-minded until he evaluates all sides of a question.
18. Has a low opinion of himself.	Thinks favorably of himself.

If your honest evaluation of yourself matches fifteen (about 80 per cent) or more of the characteristics of "Personality Two," there isn't too much room for nutritional improvement, for your nervous system is functioning at a comparatively high level.

However, should your own self-evaluations match six (33 per cent) or more of the characteristics of "Personality One," you by all means should see for yourself whether or not better nutrition will bring about a vast improvement.

The chance that it will is very great indeed.

IV Discovering Your Psychochemical Type

She would have been pretty if she hadn't been so plump. One doesn't expect to see deep-blue eyes in a setting of smooth olive skin and dark auburn hair. I could mentally trace the delicate structure of her face, now obscured by rounded pads of protruding flesh on her cheeks, her chin, her neck.

Yet she was barely thirty, far too early in life to have lost the look of being young.

Ella M. was the wife of a former patient, and all I knew in advance about her was that her husband said, "She will eat a two-pound box of chocolate-covered cherries in an evening once she gets her hands on it."

He wondered why. I also wondered why. Our joint concern led to her visit for an interview.

One of the very first things she said was, "I don't want my husband to know it, but I cry a lot when I'm alone."

She connected her "craving for sweets" with feeling depressed. Although she said she was "*never* hungry," she simply couldn't resist eating candy, cake, cookies, or "anything that's around the house that's sweet."

"When I feel very bad I simply *have* to eat something sweet," she explained, and then added, "You may not believe it, but I know my spirits pick up after I have some cookies or something."

Because of her sugar compulsion, Ella tried to avoid buying foods that might tempt her. When she got into a market, however, she couldn't always control herself. "About half the time," she admitted, "I come home with cookies or candy."

I asked her to tell me about her depressed moods. When did she cry? Did she think she had any reasons for crying?

Ella told me that almost every day after breakfast she would sit for a long time in sort of a "numb stupor," sometimes crying a little and always feeling sad and wistful. She frequently did not know what day it was, and sometimes she would suddenly realize that the month was March—not November—and that Christmas had already happened.

As the day wore on, however, Ella would gradually begin to emerge from her gloom, so that by the time her husband arrived home from work, she could meet him with a smile and actually feel somewhat cheerful for the evening.

Ella said she had no idea why she should be so depressed in the morning, yet be cheerful later in the same day, when absolutely nothing concerning her personal life was altered in any way from morning to night.

I told her that there need be no psychological reason for her depressions—that abnormal reactions such as hers most frequently result from the inability of the brain to function normally, and one of the main causes for this is wrong nutrition. I said that the first step to take in possibly finding the source of her troubles would be to analyze her food intake, and then check the way her tissues were handling the types and amounts of nutrients they were receiving.

Although taste by itself can be a very poor indicator on which to base food preferences, there are times when knowing what a person "craves to eat"—*providing his reaction to the food is favorable*—may also reveal something about his diet in general.

For example, people who eat a low-carbohydrate diet, relying mainly on fat and protein, sometimes say they are "starved for sweets"; while those whose diet is high in sugar and starch may express strong desires for salty and fatty foods.

Part of the explanation for such taste preferences may be found in the ways the cells handle different types of fuel, for the utilization of fat (and some kinds of protein) cannot take place unless sugar is also being broken down, while the complete utilization of sugar does not occur unless some fat or protein is also being burned.

I was particularly interested in finding out whether Ella's eating habits might be connected with the shifting pattern of her moods. When I asked her to tell me what she generally had for breakfast, after a moment's reflection she exclaimed, "Breakfast? Breakfast sometimes hits me like a *bomb!*"

As she described what she ate I began to get the picture, for her breakfast was indeed a heavy meal. Her husband did physical work, and wanted steak or ham and eggs with fried potatoes every day.

This diet may be excellent for someone who needs it and can handle it. But it began to look as if Ella did not need it, nor was she capable of transforming such a high fat-protein meal into energy.

Ironically, she forced this big breakfast down, she said, "because I know how important breakfast is, and I also know that if I eat what I want—like some pastry and black coffee—that the starchy, sweet food will make me gain weight."

Ella believed that the reason she was overweight was because she craved—and ate—sweets. The irony of this, however, was that she overate sweets because she tried to avoid carbohydrates almost completely!

Our blood-chemistry studies confirmed what had appeared obvious from what she had told me about her diet and the way she reacted to it. She was a slow oxidizer, unable to burn sugar fast enough to also utilize a heavy fat-protein intake. Consequently, when she ate the breakfast that was really prepared for her husband—not for her—the result was simply disastrous. The immediate psychological effect was depression, which she somewhat effectively remedied by compulsively eating sweets, so that by evening her central nervous system was again functioning almost normally.

Now, however, the vicious cycle was once more put in motion, for Ella ate another heavy meal for dinner, again skimping on starches and sugars in order to avoid gaining weight! As a result, she slept as though "drugged"—only to awaken to the still-present echoes of last night's meal. Even though she might be both depressed and somewhat nauseated upon arising, she prepared and ate another fatty meat, fried egg, and fried potato breakfast.

Although a psychotherapist had told Ella that she was a "compulsive neurotic with depressive tendencies," she was clearly nothing of the kind, if one means by this label that her craving for sweets and her depressions were both symptoms of deep-rooted psychological problems.

Ella was the unknowing victim of faulty biochemical mechanisms about which she knew nothing. The therapist who told her that she was a depressed neurotic only increased her miseries by causing her to feel guilty, by making her think that she was somehow psychologically responsible for her plight.

Ella would never have joined her husband in his heavy breakfast had she known she was a psychochemical type, a slow oxidizer, for this kind of person simply ought not to eat a heavy breakfast. Instead of having steak and eggs, a slow oxidizer may prefer to skip breakfast, drinking only juice, or perhaps black coffee, which increases the rate of sugar utilization in the brain by virtue of its caffeine content. As a matter of experience, this psychochemical type often finds that if he has had a substantial dinner the previous evening, he will think more clearly and feel much better if he doesn't eat anything for several hours after arising; or if he does eat, it will be something low in fat and high in starch and sugar, such as sweetened dry cereal and milk. A *fast* oxidizer, on the other hand, would react quickly and badly to the combination of coffee, starch, and sugar.

You may be wondering whether or not Ella could have discovered for herself that her emotional problems were connected with her patterns of eating.

The answer is not only yes, but the reason is a whole lot simpler than you might think. For Ella could easily have spotted the source of her trouble had she learned one basic fact—that unpleasant psychological reactions can directly and quickly result from wrong food choices.

I have interviewed many patients who learned this for themselves by merely putting two and two together.

Since one *can* choose a certain food on the basis of taste alone that will produce an adverse psychological reaction, one should always question a food choice which precedes any unusual emotional or mental response.

The only safeguard against making this kind of error is to establish your own psychochemical type by carefully checking *both* your food preferences and your reactions—how good, or bad, you feel after eating them.

The information on which the following questionnaire is based was obtained from research subjects whom we typed psychochemically by means of blood tests. We then found that we could equally well type new research subjects by means of an extended quiz of this kind, and confirm the results with blood tests. Write your answers on a separate sheet of paper and then compare them with the scoring table given at the end of the questionnaire.

Your Psychochemical Type

1. If I drink tea I prefer lemon with it

   _____always or very often
   _____sometimes
   _____never or rarely

2. A hamburger sandwich tastes much better with a slice of raw onion on it

   _____always or very often
   _____sometimes
   _____never or rarely

3. When I feel low I pick right up if I eat something sweet such as fruit, pastry, or candy

   _____always or very often
   _____sometimes
   _____never or rarely

4. I could enjoy eating potatoes in some form two or three times a day

   _____always or very often
   _____sometimes
   _____never or rarely

5. I could eat steak or roast beef every day and frequently more than once a day

   _____always or very often
   _____sometimes
   _____never or rarely

6. I seem to crave sour-tasting foods

_____always or very often
_____sometimes
_____never or rarely

7. Raw salad vegetables such as radishes, green onions, green peppers, and lettuce agree with me and I like to eat them

_____always or very often
_____sometimes
_____never or rarely

8. Fatty meat such as beef short ribs, spare ribs, or roast pork tastes better than very lean meat

_____always or very often
_____sometimes
_____never or rarely

9. When I feel low I feel better if I eat something salty, like nuts, potato chips, or popcorn

_____always or very often
_____sometimes
_____never or rarely

10. Sometimes I sort of drag through the day, but after a good meat dinner in the evening I begin to snap out of it

_____always or very often
_____sometimes
_____never or rarely

11. If I don't feel hungry and I eat something sweet, my appetite seems to pick up

_____always or very often
_____sometimes
_____never or rarely

12. Steak for breakfast sounds pretty good to me

_____always or very often
_____sometimes
_____never or rarely

13. I get hungry between meals and like a snack of peanuts, cheese and crackers, or maybe a hot dog

_____always or very often
_____sometimes
_____never or rarely

14. For lunch I could eat a bacon and avocado sandwich with lots of mayonnaise

_____always or very often
_____sometimes
_____never or rarely

15. I would like lettuce, cottage cheese, and fruit salad for lunch

_____always or very often
_____sometimes
_____never or rarely

16. I have a craving for something sweet

_____always or very often
_____sometimes
_____never or rarely

17. I feel better if I have some eggs with bacon or other kind of meat for breakfast

_____always or very often
_____sometimes
_____never or rarely

18. When I'm hot and thirsty I can drink a lot of something like lemonade

_____always or very often
_____sometimes
_____never or rarely

19. I like to eat raw onions

_____always or very often
_____sometimes
_____never or rarely

20. I can easily skip breakfast without getting hungry or tired

_____always or very often
_____sometimes
_____never or rarely

21. I prefer roast beef well done to roast beef cooked rare

_____always or very often
_____sometimes
_____never or rarely

22. For breakfast I feel good with something like toast and coffee

_____always or very often
_____sometimes
_____never or rarely

23. I like to drink buttermilk

_____always or very often
_____sometimes
_____never or rarely

24. Steak and lobster is my idea of a real dinner, and I could eat them together

_____always or very often
_____sometimes
_____never or rarely

25. Even after a big steak dinner I could eat a bowl of buttered popcorn

_____always or very often
_____sometimes
_____never or rarely

26. I get thirsty and drink a lot of water

_____always or very often
_____sometimes
_____never or rarely

27. I get so hungry that I have to eat something sweet between meals

_____always or very often
_____sometimes
_____never or rarely

28. When I take the cap off a jar of mustard, the smell is so sharp that it hurts my nose

_____always or very often
_____sometimes
_____never or rarely

29. I like the taste of olive oil

_____always or very often
_____sometimes
_____never or rarely

30. If I drink coffee, it seems to make me feel jumpy or jittery

_____always or very often
_____sometimes
_____never or rarely

31. I like to eat any kind of olives

_____always or very often
_____sometimes
_____never or rarely

32. I like to eat bacon

_____always or very often
_____sometimes
_____never or rarely

33. Avocados taste oily or too fat to me

_____always or very often
_____sometimes
_____never or rarely

34. I seem to need a lot of salt on my food

_____always or very often
_____sometimes
_____never or rarely

35. I would like a pat of butter added to my soft-boiled eggs

_____always or very often
_____sometimes
_____never or rarely

36. I seem to want something more to eat like cheese or nuts even after I have eaten a regular dinner

_____always or very often
_____sometimes
_____never or rarely

37. I can eat breakfast only if it is something sweet

_____always or very often
_____sometimes
_____never or rarely

38. Sweet foods like candy or cake taste too sweet to me

_____always or very often
_____sometimes
_____never or rarely

39. I like a pat of butter on a steak

_____always or very often
_____sometimes
_____never or rarely

40. Sweet things taste sweet enough to me

_____always or very often
_____sometimes
_____never or rarely

41. I prefer to eat mustard, catsup, or steak sauce on a meat patty

_____always or very often
_____sometimes
_____never or rarely

42. I seem to feel a bit weak if I haven't eaten for two or three hours
_____always or very often
_____sometimes
_____never or rarely

43. I could eat four to six pieces of bacon for breakfast
_____always or very often
_____sometimes
_____never or rarely

44. I don't like the smell of cooking food, even though it tastes all right when I eat it
_____always or very often
_____sometimes
_____never or rarely

45. I'd like broiled lamb chops for dinner
_____always or very often
_____sometimes
_____never or rarely

46. Grapefruit juice tastes very sour to me
_____always or very often
_____sometimes
_____never or rarely

47. I would like to eat baked beans with a lot of nice lean salt pork in them
_____always or very often
_____sometimes
_____never or rarely

48. If I feel a little nauseated, I feel better if I eat something salty
_____always or very often
_____sometimes
_____never or rarely

49. If I feel a little nauseated, I feel better if I eat something sour or sweet
_____always or very often
_____sometimes
_____never or rarely

50. I could drink a large glass of grapefruit or orange juice
_____always or very often
_____sometimes
_____never or rarely

51. If I eat liver, I want onions with it

_____always or very often
_____sometimes
_____never or rarely

52. I would prefer to eat bacon with fried liver

_____always or very often
_____sometimes
_____never or rarely

If you are a "slow oxidizer," you will answer "always or very often" to most (seventeen or more) of the questions numbered 1, 2, 3, 6, 7, 11, 15, 16, 18, 19, 20, 22, 23, 26, 27, 33, 37, 41, 49, 50, 51.

If you are a "fast oxidizer," you will answer "always or very often" to most (twenty-five or more) of the questions numbered 4, 5, 8, 9, 10, 12, 13, 14, 17, 21, 24, 25, 28, 29, 30, 31, 32, 34, 35, 36, 38, 39, 40, 42, 43, 44, 45, 46, 47, 48, 52.

Your food preferences and reactions are "normal," however, if you answer most (forty or more) of the questions "sometimes," or if you answer "always or very often" both to "slow oxidizer" questions (fourteen or more) and to "fast oxidizer" questions (twenty or more).

V Your Best Personality

The first thing I suggested to John Gant's wife, Agatha, after telling her that it might be possible to "increase her energy" was that she prepare a complete list of what she ate and when she ate it. Such a list might provide us with a quick glimpse of some of the more likely reasons for Mrs. Gant's introverted life-style, her lack of self-confidence, and her whole pattern of shy, fearful, and withdrawn behavior. I suspected she chose foods that decrease, rather than increase, the amount of energy being created in the tissues.

In most instances in which one is studying individuals who appear to be "medically healthy," even though they themselves do not feel that they are—no matter what the physician may say—the first place one is likely to find the reason why they feel below par is their diet.

Agatha Gant's doctor, for example, assured her that she was in "fine health," yet her whole life-style reflected a weak and ineffective personality. I found myself in for a surprise when Mrs. Gant arrived for her initial appointment. At once she asked me whether she could first "tell me something" before I looked over her diet lists.

I of course agreed, and then she said, rather firmly, "This is very important to me—I mean, that you understand. I have written down everything I can think of that I both *like* and that I can and do eat. In other words, if some food or other does not appear on my lists, then I don't *like* it, and of course I don't eat it." And then she quickly handed me a thick sheaf of note papers.

The rigid and inflexible attitude reflected in Mrs. Gant's ultimatum was just another symptom, another variety of psychochemical response, that would disappear—hopefully—with proper treatment.

So I briefly thumbed through her incredibly detailed lists of foods, thanked her for giving the matter such close attention, and assured her that I understood that her lists indicated only the things she liked and therefore the only things she would eat.

I soon discovered what I thought was a most likely cause of her psychochemical behavior. Her diet almost exactly paralleled our list of "low-performance foods" for fast oxidizers!

For example, her choices were heavily slanted toward sweets such as honey, fruit, and pastries; starches such as bread, potatoes, and spaghetti; raw salad vegetables such as green peppers, lettuce, onions, radishes, and cabbage; while her principal protein foods were milk, buttermilk, cottage cheese, yoghurt, chicken, and fish.

Since she was mainly eating the very things we ask fast oxidizers to avoid, and since she certainly did not appear to me to be functioning at her best psychological level, I would have placed a small wager—and would have won—that her blood tests would show that she was a fast oxidizer with both low blood-sugar and low blood-fat levels, who was ironically choosing the very worst possible diet, principally because she *liked* it. This case shows that people can and do choose foods which have bad effects on them, and that "liking" something is not sufficient grounds for also eating it.

When I asked Mrs. Gant at our next interview why she started the day with a tablespoon of honey in a glass of grapefruit juice—an absolute horror for a fast oxidizer!—she replied simply, "Because honey is a quick-energy food. Besides, as I told you, I like honey and grapefruit juice."

I quickly countered this "quick-energy" claim for honey by telling her that she was only partly correct. Honey indeed represents a good source of quickly absorbed and rapidly oxidized sugar. It does not, however, always represent a source of quick energy. In fact, it is one of the very worst foods a person can choose if his tissues burn sugar too rapidly, for he will have considerably less energy after eating it than he had before he ate it.

I then explained the idea of optimum nutrition, that level of nutrient intake that will support the highest level of operation of the nervous system. Since the wrong foods can actually impair brain function, one cannot hope to achieve optimum nutrition unless he both knows his own psychochemical type and also chooses the foods he eats for their performance value, and not for *any* other reason.

When I gave Mrs. Gant her vitamin-mineral formula, our list of high-performance foods for fast oxidizers, together with a chart outlining typical meals, she took one look at the menus and uttered a low "Wow!"—which I countered by saying, "It's strictly up to you."

Here is a sample of what a suggested daily breakfast looked like: no juice; ham, sausage, bacon, small steak, or ground beef patty with eggs (if desired); one-half buttered English muffin or one slice of 100 per cent whole wheat toast; Sanka (if desired).

Later her husband told me that Agatha returned home from her visit with me in a merry, almost giggling mood. "Every time she looked at the sample menus," he said, "she'd begin to laugh, and say, 'Can you just imagine *me* eating *that?*' "

Mrs. Gant probably would never have sampled even one of the suggested meals if she hadn't received a disguised gift from heaven.

She became quite ill with the flu.

It hung on and on, and she simply couldn't get her strength back. Finally, as a last resort, she decided to give the fast-oxidizer diet and the vitamin-mineral formula a try.

She later told me that when she re-read the sample menus "Somehow they didn't seem so amusing this time. In fact, some of them sounded real good."

We have already seen the kind of personality transformation that Agatha Gant experienced when her tissues were provided with the high level of nutrition they were capable of using (Chapter III, pp. 66, 67).

The shy, pensive, withdrawn Agatha became a highly motivated, confident, and successful person with many interests, many friends, and a whole new existence in the outside world that she had been hiding from all of her life.

Oddly enough, as her new personality emerged, neither she nor her husband quite grasped the meaning of what was happening.

For example, after she obtained a job her husband remarked to me, "Well, I guess Agatha's beginning to grow up, after all."

I said nothing to disillusion him, principally because past experience had shown me the futility of trying to convince someone with words alone that dramatic personality changes could result simply from improved nutrition.

In addition, however, I knew that sooner or later he would have the opportunity to get first-hand evidence for himself that Agatha was not "growing up"—as he thought—but was functioning at a higher psychological level solely because of her improved nutrition.

Then, Agatha had a setback. The firm of lawyers for whom she now worked had the custom of closing their offices for the Christmas–New Year's week, giving their employees a sort of bonus holiday vacation. Agatha took the occasion to celebrate and "live it up a little," which, incidentally, involved a return to eating all of the things she "really liked."

For example, instead of a broiled hamburger patty for breakfast, she would have buttermilk pancakes with *real* Vermont maple syrup; for lunch, a chocolate milkshake with a small cottage cheese and fruit salad; and dinner might be nothing but a big plate of spaghetti.

In addition, she baked several dozen cookies, a mince pie, and a chocolate cake, sampling these delights mid-morning, mid-afternoon, and at bedtime.

On top of all of these nutritional insults, she stopped taking her daily formula of vitamins and minerals, because, she later told me, "I just get tired of doing the same thing—like swallowing pills—day after day."

About midway through Mrs. Gant's "holiday celebration" I received a worried call from her husband. He said that he had returned from work the previous evening and had found his wife very depressed and on the verge of tears. She told him that she simply couldn't face going back to work, and asked him to call her employer and give a good excuse why she had to quit her job.

When I had a chance to see her again I asked her how in the world she could have done anything so utterly foolish. She looked a bit hurt at this, and defensively replied, "I don't suppose *you* ever make mistakes! Besides, I didn't know I was *making* a mistake. I thought I had sort of got over my old psychological problems."

One simply can't take "a day off" from sound nutrition. Whether or not one *likes* it, the heart beats on, and the liver, kidneys, and nervous system keep functioning, and their requirements simply can't be postponed.

The "holiday celebration" of Agatha Gant, which resulted in a brief return to her former introverted life-style, clearly illustrates the effect of "low-performance foods" on the personality of a fast oxidizer. Although we have already considered in general some of the biochemical reasons for this (Chapter II), it might be a good idea to review these reasons and to restate the major points in a little more detail at this time, since this will help us to understand not only why the old Agatha reappeared when she returned to her old diet, but also why her new diet–which we are going to discuss later–brought to life the new Agatha.

You perhaps recall that the sugar transported in the blood (glucose) is not only the basic fuel for all of the organs of the body, but the brain and nervous system are critically dependent upon it. The source of all energy expended by the mind is a process called cellular respiration, during which complex foods are broken down into simpler substances which are then burned (oxidized) in the individual cells of the brain. Thus, while it is customary to speak of the oxidation, or burning, of glucose, this is not to be understood literally. Glucose, as well as other foods, is transformed by the action of enzymes into a series of intermediate compounds in an interlocking, stepwise process, during which energy is formed in differing amounts at different stages in the process. In other words, energy is not derived directly from glucose but comes from several different substances, called *intermediates,* each of which ultimately has been derived from glucose.

This energy is released in "packets" which the biochemist calls ATP (adenosine triphosphate), and these packets are formed at different stages in the energy cycles, the two principal ones being represented in the vastly simplified accompanying diagram (Fig. 1). These energy cycles are called *glycolysis* and the *citric acid cycle,* respectively.

Since the packets of energy derived from the burning of fuel are released as the result of a great number of reactions, each of

FIGURE 1

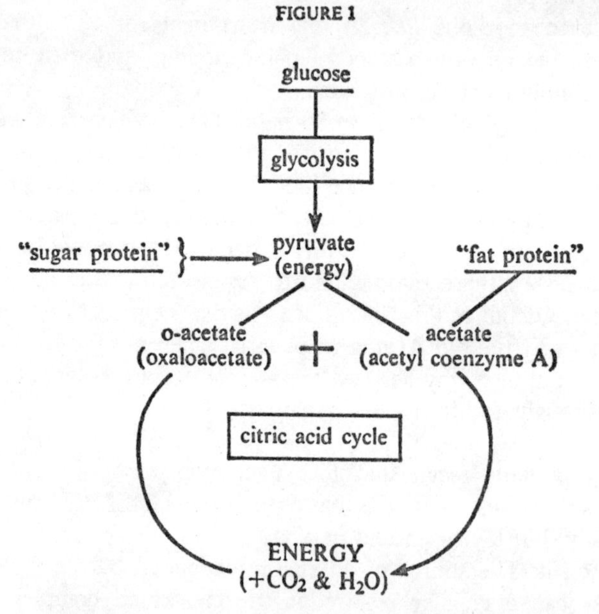

Major steps in the oxidation of sugar, protein and fat.

which depends upon the successful completion of the preceding reaction, any interference with the step-by-step breakdown of glucose in the brain results in impaired mental functioning owing to the incomplete oxidation of glucose intermediates. And one of the most frequently encountered kinds of interference is found at specific points where there are rather great demands for enzymes. For example, niacin (vitamin B_3) participates in the enzymatic breakdown of sugar at several places in the energy cycles. It is not surprising to find, therefore, that a deficiency of this critical substance has a marked effect in slowing down brain metabolism to the point of causing what appears to be mental illness. Deficiencies of other vitamins and minerals also result in a wide variety of mental and emotional disorders.

Although it is true that the nervous system relies principally upon the breakdown of glucose for energy, its ability to function properly in this regard is indirectly affected by the kinds and amounts of fuel being utilized in other tissues of the body. For example, a diet that provides disproportionately large amounts of fat in relation to sugar and starch can indirectly slow down the rate of energy formation in the brain. One of the explanations for this is that fat is burned principally in the liver, and this organ has only a limited capacity for turning it into energy. Thus the burning of excess amounts results in the formation of an oversupply of the energy-rich intermediate "acetate," which may then be carried to other tissues of the body by the bloodstream to be oxidized in the major energy-producing system of the cells, the citric acid cycle.[1] However, whether this excess acetate which has been formed from fat can be turned into energy depends upon the availability of other substances that are provided principally by the oxidation of glucose. This interlocking dependence that exists between the oxidation of different types of fuel is illustrated in Figure 2, in which glucose forms the intermediate o-acetate, which in turn can combine with the excess acetate to form citric acid, which is ultimately turned into energy.

Now if sufficient glucose is not being oxidized to provide enough o-acetate to combine with the excess acetate formed from the breakdown of a large amount of fat, the net result is a slowdown in the production of energy in the cells. The adverse psychological effects that follow are many and complex. We have seen some of them, and we will discover others in our case histories of types of mental and emotional disturbances.

[1] This statement expresses the general idea involved, although what actually happens is far more complex. However, the end result is the same. Actually, β-oxidation oxidizes fatty acids to acetate in the liver, part of which forms citric acid in the citric acid cycle, while part is converted to acetoacetic acid and passed into the blood for oxidation in other tissues, where it is reconverted to acetate and oxidized in the citric acid cycle.

FIGURE 2

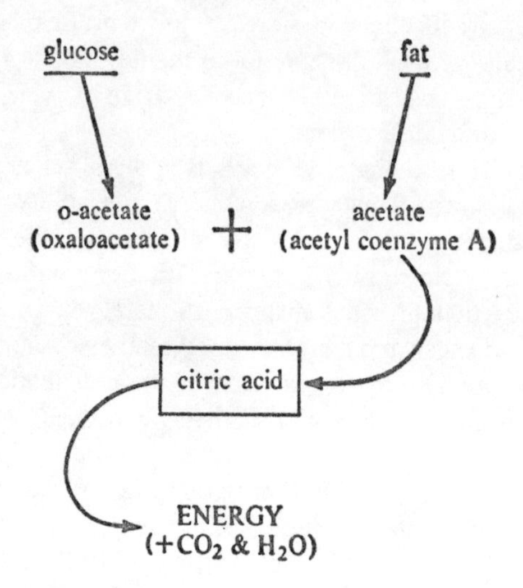

Intermediates formed from sugar and fat combine to produce energy in the citric acid cycle.

This illustration of some of the effects that can be exerted on the nervous system by biochemical reactions occurring in other tissues of the body is only one of many that may occur. However, as we have seen, our studies have indicated that there are two basic types of such nervous system reactions to the general metabolism of the body. We have just considered the first type, in which the *slow oxidation* of glucose results in abnormal mental and emotional reactions. The second type is biochemically the reverse: abnormally *fast oxidation* of glucose both in the central nervous system and in other tissues of the body results in abnormal psychological reactions.

Earlier we mentioned that any kind of interference with the step-by-step breakdown of glucose in the brain would result in impaired mental functioning. Although there are a great many individual biochemical reactions that occur in the two main energy cycles in the cells, glycolysis and the citric acid cycle, and thus consequently many possible places where trouble might develop, we have learned that there are two main points where a functional difficulty appears most likely to occur.

In the glycolytic oxidation of sugar, pyruvate is the first major intermediate that is produced (see Fig. 1). If sugar is being utilized in the formation of energy only in this series of glycolytic reactions, about 20 per cent of the total energy available in a given amount of glucose will be produced. Normally, however, the intermediate pyruvate is further oxidized to yield both o-acetate and the energy-rich compound acetate, which combine together in the citric acid cycle to produce added energy (Fig. 1). And when glucose is completely burned in both of the energy cycles in the cells, 80 per cent of the available energy is derived from the reactions in the citric acid cycle. This large amount of energy results from the complete utilization of the energy-rich intermediate acetate. However, glucose itself is a relatively poor source of acetate. Gram for gram, fat yields about three times the amount of acetate that sugar does. And although only insignificant amounts of fat are burned in the nervous system, acetate formed from the oxidation of fat in the liver appears to be utilized for energy formation in the brain. This can be clinically demonstrated when fat is severely restricted or eliminated from the diet.

Earlier we considered the example of how *excess* fat[2] in the diet could exert an adverse effect on sugar metabolism in the nervous system, through the formation of excess acetate, which, in the absence of sufficient o-acetate from sugar, could not be converted into energy (Fig. 2). A somewhat similar type of effect upon brain metabolism can result from an experimental diet that is almost fat-free, consisting mainly of carbohydrate. Although glucose breaks down to form some acetate, just as fat does, it also forms proportionally greater amounts of o-acetate. The result that follows if sugar alone is being burned is a relative deficiency of acetate to combine with the larger amount of o-acetate that is being formed. And in turn the consequences of this imbalance between excess o-acetate and insufficient acetate is the rapid use and consequent exhaustion of the supply of acetate provided by sugar

[2] When we mention fat as a source of acetate, we do not include polyunsaturated fatty acids.

alone, with a resulting lowering of the energy output of the nervous system (see Fig. 3).

Since acetate is the most important energy-producing compound in the tissues, one should not be surprised to find that rather severe personality changes can be induced by a diet very low in fat and very low in protein, the two best sources of acetate. Although individuals differ markedly in the severity of their reactions

FIGURE 3

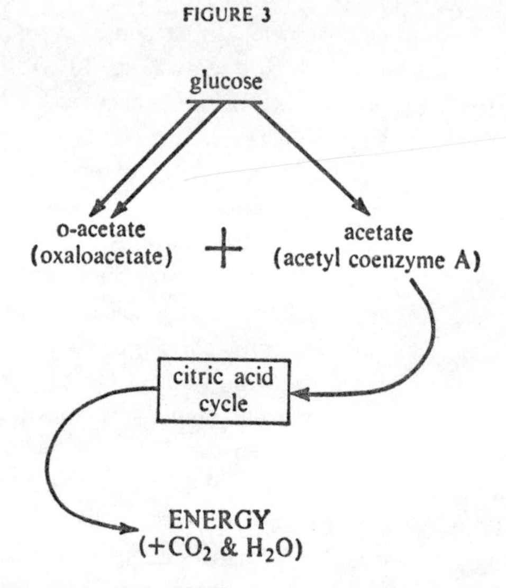

Intermediates formed from sugar combine to produce energy in the citric acid cycle.

to such a diet, all show some negative personality changes. These range from social withdrawal, anxiety, and depression, through tendencies to violence, all the way to paranoid (schizophrenic) delusions.

Earlier it was stated that any interference with the supplies of essential nutrients or with the capability of the body to utilize these to make energy at a normal rate would result in abnormal mental and emotional reactions. I have briefly described the principal processes through which the cells of the body, including the nervous system, obtain energy. In addition, I have attempted to explain two basic metabolic types of functional nervous system impairment that we have found, through many years of research, to be biochemically related to a very wide range of personality disorders. These two metabolic types we have called the slow oxidizers and the fast oxidizers. Many lines of experimental evidence indicate that slow oxidizers differ from fast oxidizers primarily in that slow oxidizers are not burning sugar rapidly enough or in sufficient quantity in the glycolytic energy cycle, while fast oxidizers are burning sugar both too fast and in too large an amount in this same energy cycle. Since the glycolytic cycle interlocks with the citric acid cycle, the normal operation of the latter depends upon the normal functioning of the former. And since about 80 per cent of the energy produced in the cells is formed in the citric acid cycle, one can see how critically important is the normal oxidation of glucose in the first stages of energy formation, glycolysis, for this ultimately regulates both the *rate* of energy release and the *amount* of energy that may be formed in the nervous system. The psychological consequences that may follow disturbances in either of these factors are many and varied, as we have already seen illustrated and will see again in greater extremes and variety in the case histories that follow.

One might think that since fast oxidizers burn sugar too rapidly while slow oxidizers do not burn it rapidly enough, it would be possible to distinguish one type from another simply by determining their before-breakfast (or "fasting") blood-sugar levels—expecting fast oxidizers to have a low level while slow oxidizers have a high one. While it is true that on the average a group of fast oxidizers will test about 20 per cent lower than slow oxidizers, there is too much individual variation to allow the use of the simple measure of blood sugar as a means of identifying individuals as to psychochemical type. The glucose tolerance test is a much more reliable indicator of impaired carbohydrate metabolism.

This test consists of administering an oral dose of glucose (usually 100 grams dissolved in 500 cubic centimeters of water flavored with lemon juice), and then measuring the level of sugar in the blood every half-hour for from three to six hours. In patients having what is called functional hypoglycemia—low blood sugar—the test dose of glucose will result in a transitory *lowering* of the amount of sugar in the blood to below the fasting level; these are fast oxidizers. On the other hand, in patients having hyperglycemia—high blood sugar—the test dose of glucose will produce a transitory abnormal elevation of the amount of sugar in the blood; these are slow oxidizers.

All medically normal persons who reveal a lowering of the blood-sugar level after a test dose of glucose and are thus fast oxidizers will also show a relative elevation of the amount of carbon dioxide plus carbonic acid in the blood. On the other hand, however—and this is important—some patients who appear to be borderline or even normal on a glucose tolerance test may still be fast oxidizers as indicated by the carbon dioxide–carbonic acid test. Consequently, if the glucose tolerance test is used by your doctor, it is wise to also have a determination of the level of dissolved carbon dioxide plus carbonic acid in having one's psychochemical type established.

In the light of this discussion of contrasting metabolic types, let us now return to Agatha Gant and take a closer look at our list of "low-performance foods" which nearly duplicates her old diet.

FAST OXIDIZER—FOODS TO USE SPARINGLY

1. *Sweets:* candy, pastries, fruit, jams, jellies, ice cream, gelatin desserts, etc.
2. *Starches:* potatoes, rice, spaghetti, macaroni, bread, crackers, cereals, etc.
3. *Salads:* lettuce, green peppers, onions, radishes, cabbage, pickles, cucumbers, etc. (celery and carrots excepted)
4. *Proteins:* milk, buttermilk, cottage cheese, eggs, fish (except herring, sardines, anchovies, tuna, salmon)
5. *Miscellany:* catchup, spicy sauces, soft drinks, coffee (decaffeinated coffee excepted), tea, beer, wine, or any other alcoholic beverage

Since the bulk of Agatha's diet was provided by items on the above list, we can now state in biochemical language why it was wrong for her: What she chose to eat was a high-carbohydrate, low-fat diet that provided too much of the glycolytic cycle intermediates pyruvate and o-acetate, and not enough of the citric acid cycle intermediate acetate to allow her to function at her full physical and psychological potential.

In addition to the imbalanced carbohydrate-fat content of her food intake, there are other characteristics of some of the foods on this list that affected her adversely. It has been mentioned that protein foods break down into simpler substances called amino acids, some of which are metabolized somewhat like sugar and some of which are handled something like fat, while a few have other metabolic routes. Thus we have seen sugar protein and fat protein, the former yielding pyruvate, the latter acetate. In addition to these characteristics of protein foods, there is another of very great importance to the energy-producing machinery of the tissues. For in addition to their amino acid content, which helps determine the amount and kind of intermediates they will yield, protein foods contain another class of substances called nucleoproteins. These are proteins which are conjugated with nucleic acids, part of which play an essential role in the energy dynamics of the cells. By far the most important of these is a purine base called adenine, which is a constituent of ATP, one of the most vital components in the body, for this compound is the principal energy carrier of the cells. Adenine also plays another important role in the cells, for it is part of the complex intermediate acetate, from which most of the energy we use is derived.

While adenine can be synthesized in the body from other substances (from CO_2, formate, aspartic acid, glycine, and glutamine), the body can also utilize the adenine contained in the diet. And for some people, the availability of dietary nucleoproteins is the difference between pervasive anxiety and forward-looking confidence, between an ineffectual personality and an attractive, successful one.

Agatha Gant was one of these. When we look at her protein intake, we find that it is not only low, but that it consists mainly of nonfat milk, buttermilk, cheese, and eggs. This is a food selection very low in nucleoproteins. Without knowing anything about it, she was inadvertently eating what is called a low-purine diet, one that yields only an insignificant amount of adenine over what the tissues can themselves synthesize, mainly from other protein (amino acids) in the diet.

Nucleoproteins, which yield the purine adenine, are found in greatest concentration in animal foods. The following list contains the best sources, ranging from 150 to 1,000 milligrams per 100 grams (about 3½ ounces) of food:

FOODS WITH HIGH PURINE CONTENT

anchovies	liver
brains	kidney
meat gravies, soups	sweetbreads
heart	mussels
herring	sardines
caviar, any type	meat extracts

The following foods contain moderate amounts of purines, ranging from 50 to 150 milligrams per 100 grams of food:

FOODS WITH MODERATE PURINE CONTENT

meat, any kind	yeast
turkey, chicken	whole-grain bread and cereals
fish	beans
shrimp, scallops	peas
oysters, crabs	mushrooms
asparagus	peanuts
cauliflower	
spinach	
lentils	

The last group contains only insignificant quantities of nucleoproteins:

FOODS WITH LOW PURINE CONTENT

all other vegetables	butter and other fats
fruit	sugars and sweets
milk	vegetable extracts, soups
cheese	
eggs	
white bread, refined cereals	

There was more than a touch of irony in the biochemical plight of Agatha Gant, for it seemed that virtually all of the principal causes of psychochemical behavior had convened in her person. Not only was she a fast oxidizer, and thus always behind in the production and utilization of acetate, and consequently never able to forge ahead mentally or emotionally under full steam, but she unwittingly enlarged this unfavorable metabolic tendency by selecting the worst possible diet, one high in sugar and starch and low in fat and protein. In addition, she possessed two other metabolic characteristics that contributed to her psychological difficulties: Her system could effectively utilize far more of the purine base adenine than her tissues were synthesizing, and she also could effectively utilize far greater amounts of certain vitamins and minerals than it was possible to obtain from her food alone, no matter how intelligently it might have been selected. Again, the first of these difficulties–her relative need for purines–she unwittingly enlarged by selecting the worst possible diet, one that offered virtually no purines at all. The second of these difficulties–her relative need for added vitamins and minerals–went unremedied because it was unrecognized.

Here is the vitamin and mineral formula she was given, to be taken every day:

Vitamin A (palmitate)	50,000	I.U.
Vitamin E	200	I.U.
Vitamin B_{12}	20	mcg.
Niacinamide	400	mg.
Calcium pantothenate	100	mg.
Vitamin C	100	mg.
Bioflavonoids	100	mg.
Choline	600	mg.
Inositol	180	mg.
Calcium	660	mg.
Phosphorus	500	mg.
Iodine	0.45	mg.
Zinc sulfate	20	mg.

Instead of relying on eggs, milk, and cheese, she was urged to eat organ meats, such as liver, as often as possible, and in any case to have servings of protein foods from the moderate- or high-purine lists *three times a day*.

Perhaps we can gain more familiarity with the basic causes of psychochemical behavior such as Agatha Gant's if we now ask whether she would have exhibited the same type of psychological withdrawal if she had been a slow rather than a fast oxidizer and had inadvertently chosen most of the correspondingly wrong foods.

To answer this question we must take another look at the two main energy-producing systems in the cells, glycolysis and the citric acid cycle (Fig. 1). We have seen that the fast oxidizer produces pyruvate and o-acetate faster than he does acetate, and is thus deprived of enjoying the full thrust of this richest energy-producing intermediate. The slow oxidizer is in virtually the same difficulty, only for exactly the reverse reasons: Although he is not behind in acetate production as is the fast oxidizer, he might just as well be, for he is not producing pyruvate and o-acetate normally from the glycolytic energy cycle necessary to convert acetate into energy in the citric acid cycle.

In either psychochemical type the same difficulty is involved: an insufficient breakdown of acetate in the citric acid cycle. The difference between them is that the fast oxidizer is not producing enough acetate; and while the slow oxidizer is producing enough, he is not able to turn it into energy.

Thus if Agatha had been a slow rather than a fast oxidizer, systematically mistaken dietary choices could equally well have contributed to produce a timid and withdrawn style of life. Such a diet of low-performance foods for a slow oxidizer would be heavily weighted with high-fat foods, protein, and particularly with foods high in purines, all of which add principally to the formation of acetate.

Here is a list of poor-performance foods for slow oxidizers:

SLOW OXIDIZER—FOODS TO USE SPARINGLY

1. *Sweets:* pastries high in fat and low in flour, such as cheese cake, tortes, Danish pastries, etc.
2. *Vegetables:* avocado, artichoke hearts, beans, peas, lentils, cauliflower, spinach, asparagus
3. *Proteins:* foods with high purine content such as liver, kidney, caviar, meat concentrates, etc. (see chart, p. 96)
4. *Fats:* lard and butter should be replaced by corn oil or safflower oil margarine
5. *Miscellany:* hard alcoholic beverages

If Agatha had been a slow oxidizer rather than a fast one, the irony of her biochemical misfortune would again be that most of the causes of psychochemical behavior had focused in her, but now with a little different twist: Instead of having a differential need for purines, unable to synthesize enough for her needs, the last thing she would need from her diet would be nucleoproteins, for these, along with fats, would cause her the most trouble.

The slow oxidizer benefits dramatically by the addition of certain vitamins and minerals to his diet, for the following are vitally concerned in the enzyme systems that participate in the breakdown of glucose to pyruvate and o-acetate, which is the weakness of the slow oxidizer. Here is the formula the slow oxidizer would take every day:

Vitamin B_1	30	mg.
Vitamin B_2	30	mg.
Vitamin B_6	30	mg.
Para-aminobenzoic acid	75	mg.
Niacin	75	mg.
Ascorbic acid	900	mg.
Vitamin D	7,500	I.U.
Potassium citrate	900	mg.
Magnesium chloride	300	mg.
Copper gluconate	0.6	mg.
Manganese oxide	30	mg.
Ferrous sulfate	200	mg.

In addition to knowing what foods to use sparingly and what foods to emphasize—the fast oxidizer using principally the foods that the slow oxidizer uses sparingly, and vice versa—both psychochemical types must use care in selecting their food to make sure that the core of their diets contains an abundant supply of protein (*not* nucleoproteins, purines, however, for slow oxidizers).

Let us review why this is so important. Although the sugar carried in the blood is the principal source of energy for both the mind and the body, very little of this important fuel can be stored for later use, only enough for a few hours if new supplies aren't forthcoming. They will be available, however, if the diet contains adequate protein, for the body can use about one-half of the protein one eats to make glucose. Protein sugar is stored in the liver as glycogen, to be converted to glucose as needed when the blood-sugar level which has been supplied directly from carbohydrate in the diet begins to run out (see Chapter II, pp. 21–24). It is the slow, gradual digestion of protein over a period of several hours that keeps a constant supply of glycogen building up in the liver to be released as blood sugar when necessary; the starch and sugar in one's actual meals are assimilated, stored, and burned much too quickly to last very long.

What constitutes an abundant supply of protein? This again is a difficult question for specialists in nutrition, because of the general confusion surrounding the concepts of "minimum," "adequate," and "optimum." I have found, however, in dealing clinically with hundreds of research subjects over almost two decades that the recommended allowances suggested by the National Research Council are sufficiently generous to meet the psychochemical needs of this group. This suggested amount is about one gram of protein for each 2.2 pounds of body weight.

Most people become a little dismayed when given this information, since they are perplexed about how to use it. Without going into the problems involved, such as the number of grams in an ounce and the percentages of grams of protein in various foods, we devised a simple rule which gives sufficiently accurate results: Simply divide your ideal weight–the weight you think you ought to weigh–by the number *fifteen.*[3] The result is the ounces in cooked weight of lean meat that will supply your protein needs per day. Lean meat includes beef, lamb, veal, pork, ham, chicken, turkey, and fish. For example, if your ideal weight is 150 pounds, you should eat at least 10 ounces of protein food from this list every day, preferably divided equally among three or more meals.

This protein rule provides a biochemical key to successful weight control through dieting, and through helping establish realistic eating habits that avert being continually hungry, overeating, and gaining weight. The pitfall in keeping slim is the wretched, miserable feeling of wanting a little something to eat–and wanting it practically all the time. This feeling is directly related to insufficient sugar in the blood, and this condition in turn is related

[3] Since the figure of fifteen as a divisor is based on an average protein content in a range of food, this method of computing one's protein intake presupposes a varied diet of fish, fowl, steaks and chops. One medium-size egg or one cup of milk may be substituted for one ounce of meat.

to both inadequate protein and inadequate carbohydrate in the diet. The only successful way one can reduce or keep from gaining weight is to maintain his blood sugar at a high enough level so he isn't hungry all the time, while at the same time limiting his caloric intake, eating less than he is burning up, the deficit being supplied by turning body stores of fat into energy.

When planning either a reducing or a weight-controlling diet perhaps the single most important thing to consider is that it is a serious mistake to think that all calories are alike and may be freely substituted for one another without taking into account the differing roles they play in the energy metabolism of the tissues. For example, sugar and starch cannot be substituted for protein, for protein supplies *continuous* fuel to keep the blood sugar high. Nor can protein be substituted for sugar and starch in the diet, for without available carbohydrate, protein cannot be converted to stored sugar (glycogen) in the liver. Finally, both fat and alcohol must be considered liabilities in relation to the sugar and starch needs of the body. Neither can substitute for sugar or for protein, and neither can be turned into energy unless sufficient sugar from dietary carbohydrate and protein are being burned.

The first thing one needs to know when planning a weight-control program is his ideal weight—that is, the weight he thinks he looks and feels his best at. It is wise to have this decided in consultation with a physician, for self-deception—thinking one is a lot slimmer than he is in fact—is known to play a large role in obesity. The weight you ought to maintain should guide both your caloric intake and the amount of protein in your diet.

Having determined ideal weight, one then determines the amount of protein he will require every day, using the simple rule mentioned above of dividing ideal weight by 15 to get the number of ounces of lean meat required daily as the core of the high-blood-sugar diet. Each ounce of this protein food will supply about 80 calories.

Let us apply this protein rule to a 5-foot 4-inch girl whose ideal weight should be 121 pounds. Her optimum protein intake will be just a little more than 8 ounces a day (121 divided by 15 = 8+). Since each ounce will contribute about 80 calories, eight ounces of meat will provide approximately 640 calories. These protein calories form the nucleus of the diet, while the total number of calories allowed per day will be determined by the rate at which one wishes to lose weight. This is determined by subtracting 500 calories a day from your normal allowance for each pound per week of weight loss.

Since the normal, nonreducing calories for this girl who should weigh 121 pounds is 2,200 per day, if she wishes to lose one pound of weight per week her reducing diet will contain 1,700 calories a day. Since the protein core will supply 640 of these, the remainder–1,060 calories–should be derived from a variety of other foods–vegetables, fruit, cereal products such as bread, sweets, and so on–largely as desired. Both the protein and the carbohydrates are *musts*. Ideally, the food in the diet other than the protein should be selected according to food groups that provide needed vitamins and minerals. Since this is generally impractical in a reducing diet because it requires more thought and effort than most persons are willing to give to it, it is wise, as a safety precaution, to supplement a reducing diet daily with a standard multivitamin and mineral formula.

It is generally agreed that it is impossible to specify an ideal diet which applies to everyone. For example, you may require still more protein (or less) than I have suggested. On the other hand, the basic facts we have been considering about the manner in which the body transforms food into energy *do* apply to everyone. But levels of energy expenditure differ, and hence what caloric reduction will be adequate for one will not be for another. In addition, individuals who are either slow or fast oxidizers will have to modify the types of foods allowed according to their own particular metabolic needs in accordance with the general suggestions given earlier.

In Chapter III we mentioned a third kind of psychochemical reactor, the suboxidizer. This type is not encountered as frequently among the emotionally disturbed as are either the slow or fast oxidizers. The suboxidizer may pass as being psychologically "normal," or may be said to have an "inadequate personality," to be "ineffective," or to be a "poor achiever." While the suboxidizer's food preferences and reactions are normal on a psychochemical quiz, their responses to a personality inventory, such as the sample given previously (pp. 69–71), may indicate that they are psychologically inadequate.

Since the suboxidizer handles carbohydrates, fats, and protein normally, what he needs to do to increase the energy output of his nervous system is to avoid casual, habitual eating practices and institute an intensive program aimed at the goal of optimum nutrition. In addition to supplementing the diet with the following suggested formula of vitamins and minerals, he should strive to maintain a high-purine intake (see p. 96) as well as a high-protein intake, following the protein allowance rule we have just been discussing.

Here is a suggested daily vitamin-mineral formula for suboxidizers:

Vitamin A (palmitate)	50,000	I.U.
Vitamin D	5,000	I.U.
Vitamin E	100	I.U.
Vitamin B_{12}	50	mcg.
Niacin	75	mg.
Niacinamide	75	mg.
Vitamin C	500	mg.
Bioflavonoids	50	mg.
Vitamin B_1	10	mg.
Vitamin B_2	10	mg.
Vitamin B_6	10	mg.
Folic acid	0.1	mg.
Biotin	20	mcg.
Calcium pantothenate	100	mg.
Para-aminobenzoic acid	100	mg.
Calcium	500	mg.
Phosphorus	500	mg.
Iodine	0.15	mg.
Magnesium chloride	100	mg.
Copper gluconate	0.3	mg.
Manganese oxide	10	mg.
Ferrous sulfate	100	mg.
Zinc sulfate	5	mg.

Many multivitamin-mineral formulas on the market approximate this combination. Check the labels: you may need to take two or three times the recommended dosage to reach this level. Health food or natural food stores are the best source.

Earlier we discussed the increased needs for massive nutritional support required by pregnancy and childbirth. This suboxidizer vitamin and mineral formula helps provide such support for those with normal metabolism, and should be taken together with the high-protein intake we have just outlined. Again, however, if one is either a fast or a slow oxidizer, the appropriate dietary suggestions for that type given earlier in this chapter should be followed.

If I were to ask you to name all of the types of fuel the body can utilize, although the reply appears obviously simple, you would probably answer incorrectly. For while carbohydrate, fat, and protein do indeed represent all the types of food we customarily think of, yet biochemically—and socially—something very important must be added: ethyl alcohol.

Although in many ways alcohol does not act as we expect food to act, since it may produce profound pathological reactions, yet from a biochemical point of view the utilization of alcohol can be looked at in the very same way that we have examined the breakdown of sugar and fat in the cells of the tissues. And while we lack a full understanding of the effects of alcohol in the system, we do know that there are two related nutritional phases to its metabolism.

First, alcohol increases the blood-sugar level by causing the liver to give up part of its stored sugar (glycogen); hence alcohol stimulates carbohydrate metabolism. Second, alcohol itself is directly broken down—principally in the liver—to produce the energy-rich intermediate acetate (acetyl coenzyme A), which is either oxidized in the citric acid cycle to produce ATP (energy) or converted to other substances such as body fat and cholesterol.

Alcohol is a rich source of acetate, ounce for ounce producing more than sugar or protein, but not quite as much as fat. In addition, however—and this point has an important bearing on its use and abuse—alcohol may be thought of as almost "instant acetate."

Let us suppose that you're physically and mentally exhausted—cold, tired, dispirited. Biochemically your cellular acetate is minimal, your blood sugar is low, and you've just about run out of ready nutritional reserves. Then someone puts a stiff drink of two ounces of 100-proof whiskey in your hand. As you sip it slowly for a few minutes, life, strength, and hope seem to push out the ache, the cold, and the despair.

If alcohol is new to you, in this moment you have had an almost unforgettable learning experience. You've been rewarded at a time and in a way that will be long remembered—consciously or unconsciously. And the next time your energy reserves are gone, and you're mentally and physically spent, you'll probably think "whiskey!" You will also have gained a personal insight into the experience behind the word, which comes from the Gaelic *usquebaugh*, meaning "water of life."

Water of life it would indeed be if the whole story of alcohol were to end with its nutritional biochemistry, and it was simply another easily utilizable and wholesome source of energy. But it is not. Every drop of alcohol burned in the tissues creates a nutritional demand for carbohydrates and for the many biochemicals that it does not by itself supply, the vitamins and minerals necessary to process it. Consequently, continued, constant, or frequent use of alcohol can lead to the depletion of cellular nutritional reserves needed for normal metabolism.

The paradox of alcohol is that while producing acetate and stimulating the breakdown of glucose, which in special circumstances results in apparent immediate physical and mental relief from stress, at the very same time this substance is a dangerous drug, both physically and psychologically.

One might think that since alcohol is metabolized in the normal nutritional pathways of the citric acid cycle, alcoholism is a nutritional disease, one that can be successfully treated by good nutrition. And indeed we have witnessed some dramatic successes using this approach. When psychological dependency has resulted from using alcohol as a substitute for food, then optimum nutrition can help erase the conditions of mental and physical fatigue which provide a stimulus to "think whiskey."

For literally speaking, if you think you "need a drink" *you don't need a drink;* you need ATP (energy) derived from acetate, through the breakdown of blood sugar, fat, and protein. If one is really well nourished his energy reserves are as high as they can be. This is why truly healthy individuals cannot tolerate alcohol:

Their cellular acetate breakdown is near maximum, and any rapid increase such as will result from a drink of whiskey may lead to headache, sweating, nausea, and possibly vomiting. In short, one's tolerance to alcohol reflects the state of one's nutritional biochemical health. The more one can drink without adverse effect the worse off he is. It is just plain utter biochemical nonsense for people to pride themselves on being able to hold their liquor, for only those in very bad shape can do so.

Unfortunately, the use of alcohol as a nutritional crutch is far from the whole story, however, for there are many reasons why people drink other than nutritional ones. For example, I had a young man tell me he was stopping his optimum diet and vitamin-mineral formula because he was "losing his taste for Scotch." He preferred the "pleasures of drinking" to the alternative I was offering of increased mental and physical functioning.

However, for those who don't *want* to drink, who find alcohol a problem rather than a continuing source of pleasure, their first goal should be to adopt an intensive nutritional program which will build them up to the point where they not only do not feel that they "need a drink"—they couldn't tolerate one without feeling ill if they drank it, amazing as that sounds.

Nutrition alone may not be able to accomplish this for individuals who have vastly overcommitted themselves to a wild and unrealistic round of daily activities. If you are one of these, take a hard look at your current life-style, and reshape it so that energy output is fully compensated for by rest, sleep, and intensive nutrition.

VI Flora Street

Miss Street was a small brunette with green eyes and a kind of "preserved" appearance. She was forty-six years old, but the way she looked made it impossible to try to guess her age. She could have passed for anything from an "old" thirty to a "young" fifty.

The way she talked made guessing her age even more difficult. Her voice was high-pitched and she spoke in a slow, deliberate manner. When she wasn't speaking she hummed an aimless melodic line, punctuated by the methodical chewing of gum. Frequently she would stop the humming and gum-chewing to emit a long, drawn-out sigh.

"I guess the reason why I'm so nervous and upset is all that fussing with my bed," she said. "I just can't hardly get any real sleep. Last night it was a little better. I only got up to iron my sheets five times."

I asked if I understood her correctly. Did she really get out of bed, remove the sheets, and then iron them? Five times?

"Yeah, that's what I said all right." She grinned a little and shifted the gum from one side of her mouth to the other. "I know it sounds kind of goofy, but I can't stand the slightest wrinkle. And once I feel one, I can't put it out of my mind and just go to sleep. Well, maybe once in a while I can forget it and go to sleep. But if I'm extra nervous I just have to get up and iron out the wrinkles."

I asked her how many times this might happen, and she said

that she could remember doing it about twenty-five times some nights.

In addition to being what she called "fussy" about her bed, she said that she was "too darn particular about everything." Sometimes when getting dressed she would remove her slip several times to iron out wrinkles that irritated her. Although her main obsessions were her sheets and her underclothes, she said she had to keep everything in the house in perfect order.

"It's really getting me down," she said rather wistfully. "I'm so worn out, I try to take naps several times a day."

Miss Street had been referred to our research program by a psychiatrist who had been giving her electroshock treatments about three months earlier. According to Miss Street, these treatments made her more ill. After those treatments failed, the psychiatrist recommended seeing a Freudian analyst. She didn't take this advice because she thought she couldn't afford it.

What the psychiatrist had in mind when he referred Miss Street to a Freudian analyst was that her bizarre obsession with her bed and her compulsion about orderliness could be understood only in terms of her childhood experiences, now long forgotten and repressed. And the particular kinds of early experiences he had in mind were severe childhood conflicts over toilet training, as well as sexual interests in parents. It was Freud's view that toilet-training conflicts regularly resulted in obsessive-compulsive neuroses in later life. In addition, however, since Miss Street was an unmarried woman who had lived alone with her father since the age of nine when her mother died, there was considerable likelihood that a Freudian analyst would expect to find a connection between a repressed infantile sexual interest in her father and her present obsession with her bed.

In other words, the Freudian would try to "make sense" out of Miss Street's bizarre behavior by uncovering the alleged "hidden meaning" behind her apparently senseless fussing with her sheets and her skirts. For to a Freudian Miss Street's behavior is really not so bizarre as it might appear to be on the surface: It makes "psychological sense"—her actions are meaningful and purposeful—once you believe you know the whole story.

However, when Miss Street was referred to me, I found reason to believe that her problems might be of psychochemical origin.

Our first clue to the possible origin of Miss Street's difficulties turned up when we found that her oxidation rate was very fast and that her tissues were burning hardly any fat at all for fuel, relying almost solely on carbohydrates. Although it is true, as we pointed out earlier, that the nervous system does not depend directly on the breakdown of fat for energy, it is indirectly affected by the amount of fat being broken down in other tissues, principally the liver. Further, patients on very low-fat diets are notably irritable, fidgety, nervous, and depressed.

We didn't have to look far to discover why Miss Street's metabolic machinery was malfunctioning, for her food intake was almost at a semistarvation level. Her diet contained hardly any fat, and her protein intake was only about one-half of what would normally be considered adequate.

For breakfast she would have toast and Sanka, or rice flakes with skim milk and Sanka; for lunch she would have a cup of milk with more toast; and for dinner she would have a small piece of meat, but the main part of the meal consisted of vegetables and dessert—pie or cake.

We gave her a food preference quiz, which turned up some rather interesting discrepancies between what Miss Street was eating and what she would prefer to eat. Here are some examples of her answers:

She said she would like to: "eat lots and lots of butter at every meal"; "eat steak three times a day"; "eat bacon or ham and eggs every morning." Miss Street was clearly a very hungry person.

When I asked her to explain these preferences, to tell me why she was eating bread and milk twice a day instead of steak, she said, "Dad kicks on the grocery bill, so I don't eat much."

It wasn't that they couldn't afford better food. Miss Street indicated this when she remarked that she didn't see why her father was so stingy, for he "had property all over town."

Miss Street's medical history revealed that as an infant she had gained very little weight during the first six months of life. She vomited everything she was fed and had to be nourished intravenously.

She reported a life-long struggle with her digestion and elimination, leading her to be almost afraid to eat for fear of becoming ill. This combination of poor digestive capability and the miserly instincts of her father probably conspired to adversely affect the normal development and functioning of her nervous system.

Needless to say, these disclosures about this patient were hardly encouraging. For it had been our experience that individuals with life-long histories of poor nutrition and assimilation responded slowly to nutritional treatment.

Miss Street turned out to be about as difficult a person to deal with as one could care to meet. She was so nervous and high-strung that at times even the sound of water boiling would upset her.

During the first six months that we worked with her, a new crisis seemed to arise several times a week. These ranged from the night songs of a mockingbird, which she asked the police to shoot because "it's driving me crazy," through abrupt changes in the weather, which upset her terribly, all the way to the real trauma of moving from a quiet, isolated house into a noisy apartment.

Every new stress resulted in a psychochemical setback, increasing the needs of her system for added nutrients of the proper kind. Despite the ups and downs, however, at the end of six months we had made significant progress. She could now sleep through almost every night without having to get out of bed and iron her sheets. She could also get dressed without having to take off her slip to iron out the wrinkles.

A few months later, when Miss Street appeared to be psychologically normal, one of our laboratory tests was interpreted to indicate that we had slowed down the rate that she was burning sugar beyond what we had intended, and that now, instead of oxidizing too fast, her oxidation rate was too slow.

This was a mistake in judgment on my part. Then, when I reversed the treatment, changing her diet and giving her a formula of vitamins and minerals to increase her oxidation rate, within one week Miss Street deteriorated completely! She was now frantically obsessed with her bed, "up twenty to twenty-five times a night, ironing sheets." She said, "I'm kind of crazy."

I reversed the treatment again, and within another week she

had returned to her former level of improvement, sleeping through the entire night without once getting up to iron her sheets.

This unintended experience clearly illustrates the nature of psychochemical behavior. It simply doesn't make any sense at all. The only "reason" Miss Street fussed with her bed and her slip was that her nervous system was not creating energy normally.

Miss Street's psychological well-being rested on a precarious biochemical foundation. It didn't take a great deal in the form of stressful activity to start the return of some of her compulsive symptoms.

At one point during our work with her we had progressed to the point where she felt good enough to obtain a job (she had never felt well enough before, even when she was a very young woman).

The result was a catastrophe. Within one month she again deteriorated completely. All of her obsessive concern with her sheets and slips returned, and the sound of a dripping water faucet made her feel like she was "going to jump clear out" of her skin.

Again, however, she recovered quickly after stopping work. This experience clearly indicated to me that although Miss Street might appear to be psychologically normal—free from obsessions, compulsions, vague fears, and depression—she would probably never be truly normal in her capacity to withstand the stresses the typical normal person undergoes without obvious trouble.

VII Jamie Pierce

The diagnosis could hardly have been worse, or hope for recovery dimmer. This tiny, shy, boyish-looking girl sitting huddled in the chair facing me had been referred to us bearing the diagnosis *schizophrenia, periodic catatonia.*

The diagnosis of schizophrenia covers a wide range of personality disorders, all involving delusions, hallucinations, and fantasy, to which the schizophrenic reacts just as though these aberrations constituted the real world. And the catatonic type of schizophrenia from which this patient suffered was marked by periods of complete psychological withdrawal and physical immobility during which she could not speak, or move—or indeed appear to recognize anyone, even her own children.

My eyes ran down the list of treatments on the photocopy of her chart that the referring psychiatrist had sent me. In addition to psychotherapy, there were repeated entries noting the administration of electroshock. She had also received several kinds of "psychic energizers," thyroid, and a wide variety of stimulants over the past four or five years.

After receiving every therapeutic aid available to her physicians, she found herself in my office as a candidate for research in mental illness.

I asked her to tell me what she believed to be her principal difficulties. When she replied I could hardly make out what she was saying; her voice was all but inaudible.

"It seems like," she said, "there are times when I can't get out of bed. And I can't move—even my tongue or lips, or open my eyes.

"Still I can hear everything that is going on around the house. The baby crying. The milkman ringing the doorbell.

"I want to see why the baby is crying, go answer the door, but I just *can't move.* You might say I'm sort of in a trance."

I asked her if she ever had advance warning, say, certain symptoms that might indicate that she was going to have another attack. Did the "trance" come on suddenly, without warning, or did it develop gradually?

She hesitated for a moment. Then, "Why do you want to know?" she asked softly. "What difference will it make?"

There is a peculiar sort of wary look one sees in the eyes of schizophrenics; Jamie had it now. Under the best of circumstances this type of patient is difficult to deal with. If she was now suspicious about a simple question, I could foresee little chance for cooperation on more difficult matters.

So I answered her question carefully, explaining that the more we knew about her symptoms the more likely it might be that we could help her.

She studied me carefully.

"If you really want to know for some *reason,*" she said hesitantly, "I don't suppose there's any harm in it."

She then told me that she did indeed have advance notice of an impending attack, that she might sort of "grope around" mentally for a day or so before losing complete contact with reality. This was good news to me, for I certainly had a reason for wanting to know whether her attacks had a sudden or a gradual onset. This patient almost literally had to be studied as two entirely different people. I needed to know what our blood tests might reveal under two entirely different conditions; first, when she felt on the verge of a period of immobility, and second, a time when she felt her very best.

I also wanted to know if she had ever noticed any relationship between what she ate and how she felt, particularly if a high-fat and high-protein diet affected her adversely. For it appeared to me that her periods of psychological withdrawal and stupor might be related to a slowdown in the rate at which her nervous system was creating energy. If this were so, the wrong foods might adversely affect her under certain circumstances.

We obtained the results of the first blood tests on Jamie Pierce the day following our initial interview; and sure enough, she was a slow oxidizer, even though when the blood sample was obtained she stated that she felt fine.

I was now faced with a dilemma. If my hypothesis concerning the biochemical origins of her illness turned out to be correct, it *might* be possible to keep her from experiencing another attack of catatonia by giving her a combination of vitamins and minerals and a special diet to help keep her oxidation rate normal. However, in such an event I would be unable to get a blood test that might tell me something about her biochemical condition when she was at her psychological worst.

Even though I really wanted such information badly, I had no alternative but to give her what I considered the appropriate treatment to increase her oxidation rate, even though it might mean that we would never get comparative tests between her worst and her best conditions. However, since her periodic attacks had been increasing in frequency, and further, since no treatment that she had received had been able to keep the attacks from recurring, I would certainly have been content even to reverse the trend and slow down the frequency of her attacks of acute illness.

The success of our treatment turned out much better than one could have hoped, however, for Mrs. Pierce experienced no periods of catatonic immobility for the next four months. This was the longest interval that she had been free from attacks for several years.

While it would be incorrect to conclude from this that her illness was under control, nevertheless this partial success indicated to me that our nutritional biochemical approach to her difficulties was fundamentally sound in principle. What I would have liked now was more information; and here again I faced the dilemma of having to keep her free from periods of acute illness, while at the same time desiring the information that such an attack might yield.

In the early fall, after Jamie had been a research patient for about six months, and during which time we had been able to maintain her on a more or less even keel psychologically, her husband decided that she was well enough to take a vacation.

I was not informed of this in advance; if I had been, I would have attempted to talk them out of it. For what Mr. Pierce had planned for a vacation was a two-week camping trip in the High Sierras. Now just about the very last thing in the universe someone like Jamie needed was a hike through the mountains by day and a sleeping bag by night. For here was a delicately balanced organism that functioned precariously even under the best of conditions.

The enemy Jamie faced at all times was stress–physical or emotional–because stress increased her needs for some of the very biochemical substances she appeared to have an unusual need for, and to which she responded favorably when she was supplied them. And while we had been able to prevent a recurrence of an acute episode of catatonia during the six months we had worked with her as a patient, the conditions under which the nutritional substances were given to her successfully at home were entirely different from the conditions she would meet on a rugged camping trip.

So I was hardly surprised when I heard what happened.

At the first sound of her voice on the telephone when she called for an appointment I knew we were in trouble.

"Is this Dr. Watson?" she asked. I could hardly hear her, and her tone seemed to suggest that she didn't even know me.

I assured her that it was I.

"You know. . . ." Her voice trailed off.

"Yes, Mrs. Pierce, what is it?"

"I don't know, but perhaps I'd better make an appointment to see you," she finally managed to say.

I didn't need to see her to get the picture. And I didn't want to waste any time on merely getting the details of what had happened.

What I wanted was a fasting blood sample at the earliest possible moment. For if she had deteriorated as badly as her voice pattern on the phone might indicate, then this could very well be the chance I had been hoping for, to see if a worsening in her psychological condition was accompanied by a slowdown in her rate of energy production.

"Mrs. Pierce," I began, "is there any chance at all of our getting a blood sample from you tomorrow morning before you have breakfast?"

She didn't answer.

"Did you hear me?" I asked.

Finally she answered. "I hear you all right," she said slowly. "It's just that I don't know. . . ."

"What don't you know?"

"Well—I guess what I mean is, what *good* will it do?"

This stunned me. It meant that her condition was very bad indeed. It also meant that I might be losing her as a research patient at just about the most critical moment possible.

"Mrs. Pierce," I said, "I obviously can't promise you that the blood test will show anything of value. But you really have no alternative! Letting us have this blood sample could be the most important thing in your life!"

My feeling of urgency reflected one bit of information she didn't know. I had been told that Mrs. Pierce was going to be committed to custodial care for life in an institution if she experienced any more attacks of catatonia. Her husband, her family, everyone concerned thought her case hopeless and helpless, and that she was destined to spend the rest of her life behind locked doors.

The following morning we obtained the blood sample.

In the late afternoon I received the laboratory report.

Comparing the data we had obtained when we made our first tests on her eight months ago, she was much worse now. Our index of her oxidation rate now was 40 per cent slower than it had been when we first tested her.

On the basis of this information we were able to prevent her from going into an episode of catatonic withdrawal by injecting directly into her bloodstream relatively high potencies of the nutritional formula she had been taking successfully in capsule form.

In thinking over my supposition that the possible metabolic causes of Jamie's illness, her periods of catatonic immobility, appeared to be connected with a very slow oxidation rate, principally a reduced capability to utilize sugar properly in the central nervous system, I decided to try to approach the problem from another angle to see whether I could get added information.

If my idea had any merit, it appeared to be almost a certainty that what she ate would also have the capability of making her ill. Unless sugar is being burned normally in the tissues, neither fat nor protein can be converted into energy at a normal rate. Consequently if one's diet under this condition of poor sugar utilization were to contain disproportionately high amounts of fat and protein, the result would be a further lowering of energy production.

The difficulty I faced here in obtaining observations from Jamie relative to the possible adverse effects of a high-fat and high-protein diet was that we had worked long and hard to improve her psychological condition; and having been relatively successful in achieving this, we had probably increased her tolerance for foods that may have been contributing to her illness in the past.

In fact the entire basis of our nutritional approach to her illness, and in general to mental illness, was simply to try to increase the functional capacity of the organism by providing substances which exerted a critical control over the mechanisms for the production of energy. And although medical textbooks might say that such energy systems are exclusively under the control of glands such as the thyroid, this is but a half-truth.

The case of Jamie Pierce is a good illustration. Well-meaning physicians who had tried to treat her illness in the past most frequently started by administering thyroid substance. And every time she received it, she told me, it made her much more ill. Indeed, she said that on one occasion an injection of thyroid had put her in a "coma."

I was not surprised to hear this from her, for I had heard similar reports from many patients whom we had classified as having metabolic problems similar to Jamie's. The reason for this untoward reaction is that in general the net effect of thyroid hormones is to produce hyperglycemia—the very *last* thing a slow oxidizer needs, since his blood sugar is already too high and he is having trouble burning it.

Although we had Jamie now to the point where the diagnosis of schizophrenia, periodic catatonia, which she bore when she was referred to us, was no longer applicable, and the specter of lifelong confinement in an institution appeared to be gone, she still had one problem that bothered me. About one week before the beginning of her menstrual period she would become very nervous and tense, and sometimes depressed.

Interestingly enough, however, as the symptoms of her periodic episodes of catatonia left her, the premenstrual difficulties also improved. In fact, I noted that there probably was some connection between the two when she had first reported to me in our initial interview that she "predictably missed her period every other month," but when she began to improve biochemically she also stopped missing periods.

Now if there was a connection between the metabolic disorder which we believed to have caused her mental symptoms and the missing of periods—as well as the current episodes of premenstrual tension—then it occurred to me that I still might be able to test my idea that a low-carbohydrate, high-fat, and high-protein diet might have an adverse effect on her.

I included here the category of high-protein foods along with the fats for at least two reasons. First, most protein foods are also high-fat foods, and second, a significant part of protein (the so-called ketogenic amino acids) is handled in the tissues somewhat as fats are.

What my idea involved was first to ask Jamie to go on a diet that contained as little fat as possible, while using nonfat milk as the only source of protein, and even this was to be kept at the minimum she required to maintain her protein balance. She was to begin this diet when she first noticed symptoms of premenstrual tension.

Now if indeed her monthly tension, depression, and nervousness were related to the same kind of metabolic difficulty that had appeared to bring on her acute attacks of catatonia, then such a diet ought to have the effect of helping relieve her premenstrual symptoms. Or so it seemed to me.

At any rate, Jamie was agreeable to undertaking this program, although she appeared to be extremely skeptical that anything so simple as the food she might or might not eat could exert any significant effect on her periods of tension, much less on her depression.

When she called to report how she was getting along with the diet, she seemed genuinely surprised.

"I really can't believe it!" she said.

"Can't believe what?"

"Well, here I am only a few days away from when my period is supposed to start, and I don't feel a thing!"

I suppose that her surprise–amounting to disbelief–really stemmed from the fact that she, like most people, had never considered mere food to be anything more than something you either liked or disliked, wanted or didn't want.

"Perhaps you don't feel a thing, as you say, because you're going to miss your period this month," I replied.

"No, I really don't think so, for there are other signs. I just don't feel nervous or tense."

At this point I couldn't resist asking her to do something which might give me some more information, even though it might also bring some discomfort.

"You know," I said, "I really would like to be sure about this. I'd like to see what might happen if you *reversed* the diet temporarily, to see whether or not you might feel any different."

I went on to point out how difficult it was to obtain reliable information in this kind of matter, and that for all either of us knew, the diet of high sugar and starch, low fat and protein, had little, if any, effect on the way she now felt.

On the other hand, I said, if we were to suddenly reverse the diet and obtain a different reaction, that might give us a little more confidence in our estimate of what was going on.

She agreed to the experiment. But I would never have suggested it had I had any idea of what was going to happen.

Several days later she called me to report. When I heard her voice I had the information I had been after; it was almost the old Jamie, the sick Jamie.

But not quite.

She was not too far regressed to report rather clearly that after several days of eating "very heavy" meals, she capped the experiment with an unusually large roast chicken dinner on Saturday night.

She was unable to get out of bed all day Sunday!

Further, she said she felt just like she "was in a sort of trance" —just the way she used to feel when a period of catatonic immobility was developing.

This told me clearly what I wanted to know. For these experiences of Jamie's were so sharply in contrast that I simply had to take them seriously. First she had reported a very good reaction to the diet of high sugar and starch, low fat and protein. Not only was this good reaction immediately erased when she changed to a low-carbohydrate, high-fat, and high-protein diet, but she also had precipitated an acute attack of illness, the first in many months.

Jamie's experiences with these different diets had been just about what I had been led to suspect on the basis of the contrasting blood tests we had obtained on her when she was mentally ill and when she was free of such illness.

Everything appeared to be tied together, particularly the very large fact that we had been able to prevent her from having attacks of periodic catatonia. And we had done this by giving her nutritional biochemicals, certain vitamins and minerals (formula on p. 99), which were known to act in the tissues as parts of enzymes concerned with the breakdown of sugar, fat, and protein.

The very marked reactions which Jamie had experienced by simply altering the kinds and amounts of food in her diet had a profound effect on her attitude toward what heretofore she had taken for granted. And now that her attention was directed to the possible psychological consequences of dietary changes, she recalled that in the past she had lived "for days at a time, it seemed," on little but orange juice. She had never thought about this other than to think how really good it tasted to her.

But now she recalled that whenever she had felt "out of touch with the world," she would drink orange juice all day, "to keep going."

When I showed her the comparative blood test results we had obtained when she was stuporous and ill and when she felt normal, and explained what I thought the significance was, she seemed to grasp the reason she might have gone for the orange juice as a source of sugar at a time when its lack might very well have pushed her into a period of illness.

"You know," she said, "if anyone had ever tried to tell me that I was perhaps just one meal, the *wrong* one, away from a mental hospital, I would have known for sure that someone was crazy, and it wouldn't have been me!"

I laughed, pointing out that this wasn't quite accurate, for it might take an unusual sequence of so-called "wrong meals" to produce such a result.

"If what you're saying is that there is nothing wrong with my diet but something wrong with me," she wanted to know, "have you any idea how I got this way?"

I told her that if she was asking me whether I could tell her how she became almost incapable of handling certain foods like fat in her diet because she didn't burn sugar fast enough, the answer was no. For almost every day I see a patient that has the *reverse* problem; if he indulges in sugar and starch to hardly any degree, he begins to feel like he's going to lose his mind.

Through the combination of taking the vitamin-mineral formula and watching her diet carefully, we were able to virtually eliminate Jamie's periods of premenstrual tension. But not quite. If unusual stresses developed during the month, she might have a difficult week or so just before her period was due.

This appeared to me to be a problem that we ought to try to eliminate entirely. I didn't like the prospect of having to severely restrict her diet for part of each month, indefinitely.

So I suggested to Jamie that she see an endocrinologist whom I knew and who had been unusually successful in treating this particular problem with hormones.

Her initial reaction to my proposal was a flat "no," because she said that she had been through that kind of treatment before, when she was missing periods, without success. However, I finally convinced her that she ought to take my advice in this matter, for she was not quite the same person now, since she was no longer mentally ill and she was no longer missing periods.

Within the span of four months, the tensions, nervousness, and depression that had marked her premenstrual week were all but eliminated by the androgen-estrogen treatments given to her by the endocrinologist.

She was now able to eat a normally balanced diet, and except for the normal ups and downs that everyone experiences in trying to cope with children, spouse, house payments, and the like, Jamie's real difficulties appeared to be in the past.

But one never knows, and one always wonders what the future may turn up.

Almost five years later I received a telephone call from Jamie. Since I had last seen her, she had moved to New York, and she was now back in town for a brief visit.

I asked her to come to my office, for here was a relatively rare opportunity to follow up a patient, to see what the long-term consequences of the treatment had been.

I need only relate a fragment of our conversation. It tells the story of Jamie Pierce.

"You know," she said, "when I tell people that I used to be a catatonic, that I used to have schizophrenia, they just laugh! I get so mad, but they won't believe me!"

I said nothing, for the thought depressed me.

The specter of all the other Jamies in the world loomed before me.

"Dr. Watson," she said, "when are you going to *do something* about it?"

VIII Face to Face with a Hostile Critic

One late Friday afternoon I was entertaining in my laboratory a research professor from a famous nearby technical institute. I will call him Peter Cameron. He was English, and he enjoyed the distinction of possessing three degrees: M.D., D.Sc., and Ph.D.

These titles of course represent a considerable achievement of erudition; since I had never met him before and since he had come to visit me at the urging of a graduate student who was interested in our research, I was more than a little eager to appear knowledgeable and competent.

But I almost didn't make it.

For we had barely exchanged a few social pleasantries when the red emergency light began flashing on the telephone. I excused myself and took the call.

"It's Dr. Warren, and she says it's an emergency!" said the operator.

Dr. Warren sounded very anxious. "I hate to bother you with this, but a friend of mine has just had a psychotic break!"

Dr. Warren had served as a consultant in our research program in her specialty as a physiological psychologist, and she knew as well as I that this sort of thing demanded the immediate attention of a physician and a psychiatrist.

"I'm sorry to hear that," I said, "but what has this got to do with me? What you need is medical help, not a conversation with someone who does research."

"Yes, I know all about that, but this situation is a little bit unusual. The family will not allow a psychiatric consultation."

Dr. Warren said she had known this family of three unmarried sisters for many years. They were all just past middle age and lived together in an old mansion in a formerly fashionable part of town.

This day, just after lunch, the youngest of them, Virginia, had hurriedly gone to her room upstairs and slammed the door. The next thing they knew, furniture began flying out the upstairs window, accompanied by an incredible commotion of breaking glass, loud cracking noises like cabinets being smashed, and the general hair-raising hubbub of someone going berserk.

I asked Dr. Warren whether or not the family had called a physician, even though they might not be persuaded to call a psychiatrist. Dr. Warren knew, of course, that a family doctor could probably handle the agitation with an injection of Thorazine or some similar tranquilizer.

"No," she said, "the girls are afraid that if they do, Virginia will be put in a mental hospital. They simply won't take the chance of this happening. They've been through it before. They'll just wait it out."

"Wait it out!"

"Yes. They think that she'll exhaust herself in a few days, and after that she'll act funny for a while, and then gradually get back to acting all right."

"Well," I said, "if that's their plan, why have you called me? You must know that there is absolutely nothing I can do in a situation of this kind."

What Dr. Warren said next really took me by surprise. She asked, "Would you send me some of the experimental formulae you are using in your current research?"

Suddenly I remembered my guest, Dr. Cameron. I had all but forgotten his presence. I made a half-turn in my chair away from the telephone to find Dr. Cameron staring at me with an intent, interested, and puzzled look.

He had probably heard both ends of the conversation, for Dr. Warren was speaking loudly. I was more than a little embarrassed by what must have been going on in his mind. Of all the impossible times in the world to be confronted by such a bizarre situation! But right now I couldn't worry about what his reaction might be.

"You surely don't know what you're asking," I told Dr. Warren. I hardly knew where to begin with my list of objections to letting her try an experimental procedure on her disturbed friend.

"In the first place," I began, "there's the matter of medical responsibility."

Dr. Warren brushed this aside by saying that the sisters knew someone whom they might persuade to take the responsibility for the patient.

I asked, "Do you mean to tell me that this physician would approve even tacitly of the use of an experimental procedure he's never even heard of?"

"Well," Dr. Warren said, with a note of impatience, "you don't understand the whole situation. The girls won't take drugs, for religious reasons; but they don't object to what I've told them of your methods."

"If they won't take drugs, how come they know a physician at all, much less one who might cooperate in this situation?"

Dr. Warren replied that the doctor was a female general practitioner whom the sisters had known for some thirty years and who understood the girls' attitude toward medicine. She added, apologetically, "They call her only as a last resort."

I reminded Dr. Warren of another, practically insurmountable, obstacle to her plan to employ our research methods on her psychotic acquaintance. "Suppose," I told her, "that you could get the sisters' doctor friend to go along with you. And even suppose further that I could obtain the permission of our medical director to let you try this experimental procedure—which, by the way, is rather unlikely. Even granting the solution of these difficulties, I'm afraid I still can't help you."

"You *can't!*" She sounded utterly dismayed.

I then explained to Dr. Warren that before I could supply her with the materials for the treatment I would have to have blood tests made on the patient. Without the information that the tests *might* supply, I would have no idea how to proceed. I also reminded Dr. Warren that without such biochemical information, no treatment could be undertaken, since it was entirely possible that the patient could be made more ill by administering the wrong treatment.

"Well," Dr. Warren replied, "would you mind if I checked with the sisters and with their doctor and called you back?"

I agreed, reasonably certain that this would be the end of the matter—they wouldn't be able to get the patient to the laboratory for an early morning fasting blood test, and our medical director would never permit us to go ahead. I now became acutely aware of the presence of Dr. Cameron.

"You know, I'm really sorry for this long interruption," I began.

"Think *nothing* of it. As a matter of fact," he continued, "I must apologize; but I couldn't help hearing, and I was quite fascinated by every bit of it."

No doubt. And I knew what was coming next, for I had mentioned the necessity for having blood tests made as a condition for treatment.

I had no desire to discuss these tests with Dr. Cameron. They were still in the exploratory research stage; and even more important, they could by no means be construed to be a diagnostic procedure to identify mental illness.

Dr. Cameron continued: "I must admit to being a bit curious about whatever tests of such critical importance to you could be."

I ran down the list of tests we were currently using, which contained about twenty items, all old stuff and all too familiar, things such as blood glucose, total lipids (fats), red and white blood cells, protein-bound iodine, and so on.

He was puzzled about the tests I mentioned—why would we spend time and money on what appeared to be futile—futile because no blood tests of any kind had ever been discovered to be of value in discriminating mental illness?

It was an awkward moment for both of us. I didn't want to appear to be an idiot, and he was too polite to accuse me of being one. Just as I was about to try to change the direction of the conversation, the telephone rang again. Not only was I *not* saved by the bell; I was thereby forced to disclose the very thing I had the least intention of mentioning.

The call was from the head of the clinical laboratory, informing me that he had been asked by our medical director to make a house call at seven thirty the next morning—the sisters! He was checking with me to find out what tests we wanted performed on the blood sample.

I started to explode.

"Really," the lab director countered, "I don't know a thing about this except that I've been on the phone for at least a half-hour with three different doctors. Dr. Warren told me that you said that if the medical director approves, to arrange for a residence call to this patient."

It was too late to back out. I suppose I *had* given my implicit agreement to go ahead with Dr. Warren and let them use our experimental treatment if the blood test could be made and if the two physicians approved.

"What tests are we supposed to run on the sample?" the lab director asked again. "I should tell you that if the patient is agitated, we might not even get a sample of blood at all. So we'd better plan on as few tests as possible, because we might not have enough blood to perform all of the regular tests."

"Well," I replied, "in case you can obtain only a small sample, you had better just check the plasma pH and the total carbon dioxide content."

I was watching Dr. Cameron as I said this. I was almost expecting him to wince at the mention of pH and CO_2 content, for I could well imagine my own reaction under similar circumstances. Here we have a frenzied maiden lady barricaded in her bedroom, demolishing everything that yields to her newfound strength. The corrective measures require a simple measure of the acid-base balance of the blood, to be followed by some vitamin and mineral capsules!

"Dr. Cameron," I began, "I wouldn't like you to believe that this is a typical day for us." I tried to smile but I couldn't.

He merely nodded.

His reflective silence seemed to ask for some further explanation of the episode.

I told him that I would like very much to explain why I had asked for tests on both the hydrogen ion concentration (the pH) and the carbon dioxide content of the blood.

"You know," I began, "it is widely recognized that some kinds of mental illness result solely from the absence of certain necessary biochemicals in the diet. The most familiar example is the mental derangement that comes with pellagra, owing to insufficient niacin.

"On the other hand, not too many of us are aware that a mere reduction in calories—especially those normally obtained from fat in the diet—say, as found in starvation or in reducing regimens, can also cause mental and emotional disturbances."

"Really?" Dr. Cameron asked. "I hadn't heard about reducing diets in this connection."

"Well," I continued, "I just mentioned the diets in passing. What I'm really interested in is something that happened many years ago when I and some colleagues began investigating the relation between nutritional intake and psychopathology.

"We began this research with the rather simple-minded assumption that we might find significant deficiencies in the critical nutrients among mentally ill people.

"We did find some of these. But we also found something that we were totally unprepared for. We found that not only could the *absence* of certain nutritional factors vitally impair mental health, but that the *excess* of some of these very same factors in certain persons could also vitally impair mental health."

I paused to let that sink in, for I had found that few persons trained in the basic principles of physiological chemistry were prepared to accept these findings without argument.

Dr. Cameron was no exception.

He said, "I find that hard to accept. I've never heard or read anything of the sort." His tone was authoritative.

"Well," I rejoined quickly, "you'd believe it if you ever found yourself making your patients more emotionally disturbed by administering some 'simple' nutritional substance they didn't need and couldn't handle."

"Do you mean to say this is something that might happen frequently?"

"My principal concern with any research patient is first to see that it *doesn't* happen. And," I continued, "take my word for it. We've learned this the hard way, by carefully screening every vitamin, mineral, and other dietary substance we could for its possible positive or negative effects in a given type of patient."

Dr. Cameron didn't seem to like what I was telling him, and he was slow to comment.

"Well," he said finally, adopting the authoritative tone again, "I think that what you might be saying is that you're evoking allergic responses or something of the sort by using large amounts of vitamins and such which the body was never designed to handle in the first place."

The conversation was beginning to follow a grimly familiar pattern. Right now I had no wish to argue the matter further.

"Forget about the vitamins," I said to him. "They're only part of the picture. I'm also talking about beefsteak, olive oil, cinnamon candy–you name it. It could be anything at all. Under certain circumstances in a certain person, you may have trouble.

"And," I continued, "if we had the time, I believe I could offer you a pretty good explanation, in the language you understand–the language of the mechanisms for energy release in the processes of intermediary metabolism.

"Suppose you grant that we face the possibility that something we give a patient might inadvertently make him more ill. Since this is absolutely the last thing anyone would desire, our first concern must be that it be prevented."

"Reasonable enough, I would say," agreed Dr. Cameron.

"Now, perhaps you recall the tests I told you we were performing on our research patients. At the time you seemed puzzled about our checking such obvious things as thyroid function, blood count, blood sugar and fat, and all the rest. Well, we have been trying to find something, *some* measure–anything at all–that we can correlate with both the patient's favorable response to treatment and his possible unfavorable response."

This was a simple statement of a purely empirical procedure that Dr. Cameron could understand and accept in principle.

"You think you have found a significant relationship between the kind of treatment you give and the pH and the CO_2 content of the blood? I must say this is curious. Perhaps you are mistaken."

"As far as being mistaken is concerned," I replied, "in this kind of research one frequently reaches the conviction that he was *born* mistaken. However, in this particular matter I do feel that we may be partly wrong, and possibly mainly right—but this is not the time to explore the complexities involved.

"Let me make a suggestion. We are going to have a measure of the plasma pH and the total carbon dioxide content on this agitated woman. Why don't you phone me tomorrow afternoon and let me tell you what we have found and what we propose to do on the basis of the test results?"

Instead of phoning me the next day, Dr. Cameron paid me another visit to ask about the results of the tests.

"Well, what did you find?" Dr. Cameron asked.

The violent outburst that had occurred in Virginia's bedroom had been followed by a period of lethargy during which she seemed not to recognize anybody or anything. The blood sample was obtained without difficulty.

"By any standards," I said, "the blood was far from normal. The pH was 7.55, and on the total carbon dioxide we computed the base to be 17.0 and the dissolved CO_2 to be 0.60.

"I'm sure, Dr. Cameron, that you're aware this last figure is less than half the amount of dissolved carbon dioxide one would expect to find in a normal healthy adult."

"Yes—by some standards," Dr. Cameron said.

He paused for some time. When he spoke again, his tone and manner had changed.

"Tell me," he asked, "just what do you make of this? How do you interpret these numbers?"

To me this was the very devil of a question. As with almost any standard measure employed in clinical biochemistry, what the numbers might "mean" would depend on other information. It would be impossible to state decisively what they meant without knowing what they *didn't* mean.

I had a feeling that what I was going to hear next from Dr. Cameron was a recital of textbook interpretations of what the numbers "meant." His authoritarian manner of judging and speaking was beginning to irritate me. So I decided I'd feed him his textbook interpretations before he could call my attention to the fact that I was overlooking what every "authority" knew was the case.

"Well," I said deliberately, "when you want to know how I

interpret these abnormal test values, I cannot give you a concise answer."

"What do you mean by that?" he inquired. "After all, you ordered just these tests run on a psychotic patient, and no others. You must have had a definite reason for it."

"Yes, to be sure. But all I can assert right now is that they *are* abnormal. For example, the patient may have a brain tumor which is stimulating the respiratory center to cause hyperventilation, so that we find the carbon dioxide in the blood lowered due to rapid breathing. On the other hand, she may have been taking large doses of aspirin for arthritis—which could also cause her to blow off carbon dioxide in hyperventilation.

"In addition, there is always the possibility that her violence in smashing up the place was really a phase of delirium which might accompany encephalitis."

"Now, really," Dr. Cameron said, "you simply can't be serious about this. You don't mean to tell me that you ordered these tests as a catchall to spot a dozen or more possibilities!"

Ignoring his comment I continued, "In addition to the things I've already mentioned, there are other possibilities; for example, the patient may have been suffering from an anxiety neurosis, which was making her breathe too fast."

"Well," said Dr. Cameron, with a sort of I-told-you-so tone in his voice, "that's a bit more like it!"

I shook my head vigorously. "I don't believe that there is one chance in a million that any of the things I've mentioned has any bearing whatever on either the condition of the patient or on the abnormal values that we obtained from a sample of her blood."

"Then why did you mention them at all?" Dr. Cameron wanted to know.

"Simply to clear the air and to keep you from having to do it for me."

"Now, really, you know," Dr. Cameron began, "one just doesn't dismiss these things you've ticked off as mere one-in-a-million shots. Just suppose this lady has a tumor on the brain? What then?"

"Let me say first, Dr. Cameron," I replied, "that this particular case is something unique to me. You recall that these sisters do not accept medicine because of religious convictions. Under ordinary circumstances a physician would have been summoned, which would lead to the employment of neurological techniques if necessary to rule out the possibility of a tumor on the brain.

"For the typical research patient who participates in our studies, every effort is made to rule out possible pathologies by medical screening. Every possible explanation of the abnormal findings has to be eliminated before I have anything whatever to do with the patient."

"I see," said Dr. Cameron. "Then just how *do* you interpret these numbers?"

"Well, let me put it this way: As you well know, exploratory research of the kind we're doing generally is guided by a working hypothesis–an interpretive basis–which we use to try to understand and explain what we think is going on.

"In this sense let us say that I'm going to act on the idea that this psychotic woman has a depressed oxidation rate. That is to say, she is not burning fuel normally in her tissues, particularly the nervous system."

"Perhaps what you're saying is a bit too general for me to be sure I understand," Dr. Cameron said.

"Let me put it in the simplest way I can. We all know that the end products of all of the substances which the body may use as fuel–fats, sugars, starches, and part of the protein–are two simple substances: carbon dioxide and water.

"An analogy is the familiar one that the smoke from the burning of leaves, grass, and wood is something like the carbon dioxide from the body's use of fat, carbohydrate, and protein.

"Now since the level of dissolved carbon dioxide carried in the blood of our patient was less than one-half of what we would expect to find in a normal person, I'm going to entertain the idea that this resulted from a 'slowly burning fire'–an *indication* that she may not be oxidizing fuel properly in her tissues, particularly carbohydrates, and this is affecting her nervous system.

"I am therefore going to supply Dr. Warren with some capsules containing certain vitamins and minerals which we know to be necessary for the normal oxidation of fuel–mainly glucose–in the cells of the tissues."

Dr. Cameron shifted uneasily in his chair. "If I may make one small interruption here," he interposed. "If as a matter of fact the patient's oxidation rate *is* slow, as you suggest, then obviously what she needs is thyroid or possibly some other hormone, such as insulin."

"Dr. Cameron," I asked, "do you really believe that if a person happened to need a certain vitamin like thiamine in order to synthesize a critically important enzyme on which the ultimate oxidation of glucose depended, that you could *substitute* a grain of thyroid?"

I was beginning to feel exasperated, and I'm afraid I showed it. It wasn't just Dr. Cameron I was reacting to, but to the many suggestions that had reprovingly been offered to me by highly trained persons who ought to have known better.

"Well," Dr. Cameron said apologetically, "I didn't mean quite what you seem to think I meant. Certainly I couldn't substitute thyroid for an enzyme. What I meant is that the patient was far more likely to require thyroid."

I then told Dr. Cameron that we checked the thyroid function as a matter of routine in all of our patients, extending over a period of several years, and we had never found one abnormal result that reflected the condition of the patient.

"Is that right?" he asked, his tone suggesting disbelief.

I thought it was long past the time to put an end to our futile and fruitless conversation.

I said, "I'll tell you what. Dr. Warren already has the capsules. I'll check the progress of the patient with her, and in a few days or weeks we'll try to get another blood sample. We'll get the blood whenever those who are supervising and observing the patient believe she is her 'normal' self again.

"I'll wager you a hundred to one that when she is normal, the level of dissolved carbon dioxide in her blood will be *double* what it was on the first test when she was psychotic."

Dr. Cameron laughed.

Two days later I received a call from Dr. Warren.

"I just called to thank you for your help," she said.

"What are you thanking me about?" I asked.

"Well, of course, for your help with my upset friend."

"I must say you have a light touch in dealing with a matter as serious as this. Tell me what happened!"

Dr. Warren's matter-of-fact way of thanking me suggested that she considered this kind of situation to be an everyday occurrence in my life, with the issue never in doubt.

Dr. Warren laughed. "You'll have to forgive me. I've been so close to this affair that I just sort of assumed you were also.

"Well, Virginia had three doses of the capsules you gave me on the day the blood sample was taken. I wasn't there that evening, but the sisters say they felt she started to come out of it by bedtime. The following morning she was noticeably more alert and more at ease, and had a fair appetite. She's about the same today, still in sort of a daze, but not noticeably disturbed and not really apathetic."

"Well, this is certainly good news," I told Dr. Warren.

"How long do you think," she asked, "it will take to return her to something resembling her normal self?"

Here again Dr. Warren simply seemed to take for granted that a handful of our experimental pills would turn the trick, an assumption I by no means shared.

I told Dr. Warren that I hadn't the faintest idea; all we could do was wait and see. I asked her to keep in close touch with the patient; and when the sisters agreed that Virginia appeared to be about normal again, I wanted to know so that we could obtain another blood sample for purposes of comparison.

It was about three weeks later that we were able to repeat the blood tests on Virginia.

Recalling my hasty 100-to-1 wager with Dr. Cameron that when the patient was normal the dissolved carbon dioxide level in her blood would be doubled, I was almost afraid to read the report from the laboratory.

As it turned out, I would have lost the wager.

But not by much.

The first blood sample we had obtained from Virginia when she was severely disturbed mentally had shown a pH of 7.55, a plasma bicarbonate of 17.0, while the dissolved carbon dioxide was 0.60.

The results obtained from the new blood sample when she was

"normal" showed a pH of 7.42, a bicarbonate of 24.0, and a dissolved carbon dioxide of 1.14.

It was only a 90 per cent increase. But I was elated with this result, and anxious to confront Dr. Cameron with it. A large part of my motive here, I must admit, was personal—to try to reconstruct my own image as knowledgeable and competent.

Three days later Dr. Cameron met me for lunch at the University Club. We had both been invited by our medical director, and it turned out to be a pleasant social occasion with little technical discussion of any kind. After lunch Dr. Cameron returned with me to the laboratory.

"I hope you've forgotten my rash offer to wager a hundred to one that if the disturbed sister regained her normal composure we would also find that the dissolved CO_2 level in her blood would have doubled," I began.

"Well, of course, I thought you really must have been joking," he replied.

I handed him copies of both reports from the clinical lab.

"You can see that I would have lost the wager, since the increase was *only ninety per cent.*"

Dr. Cameron was furious.

"Do you mean to tell me that you really believe that these last tests have anything to do with the improved psychological condition of this patient?"

I was silent.

"And perhaps you also believe"—and now his tone turned to sarcasm—"that the vitamin and mineral capsules you sent—which she may or *may not* have taken—were the reason for this increase in CO_2?"

"Well," I said slowly, "let's take one thing at a time.

"First, I most certainly *do* believe that if we have an abnormally low or high reading on this variable, while at the same time the patient is otherwise physically well but psychologically abnormal, then and only then would I connect the CO_2 reading with the psychological state of the patient."

I paused to let him think that over.

Then I continued. "Let me put this another way. I do not believe—and I have never intimated—that we have a test for mental illness. I would presume that one could obtain quite abnormal values on the measures we are discussing among people who are more or less 'normal' psychologically. I really don't know about this, except to say that there are individual differences in response to greatly increased or decreased oxidation rates—some people are more affected than others.

"As for your second question, as to whether or not I believe the capsules I gave to Dr. Warren were the cause of the observed change in the patient, you may remember, Dr. Cameron, that I did not offer to wager you that our experimental treatment would bring about a change in the patient. What I said, and I was quite careful in my choice of words, was that when the patient is normal, the CO_2 will have doubled.

"Now I obviously have very little information on this particular patient. There might have been any number of things influencing her that I know nothing about. But I will say this: *If* the patient is similar to those we have under study—and the only change in her regimen was our intervening treatment—then there is no doubt in my mind that the capsules I gave to Dr. Warren, some of which she observed the patient taking and others she was assured the patient took, were responsible for the increase in the CO_2 that we measured."

There was a long pause. When Dr. Cameron spoke, his manner and tone had changed from indignation to indifference. "I don't suppose that anyone can prevent you from believing what you want to."

It suddenly occurred to me what the trouble might be. I remembered that he had said he was an endocrinologist, and that his research interests were in thyroid hormones and diabetes. It couldn't have been worse, for here I was entering his domain and challenging his articles of faith—among them the belief that hormones such as thyroid and insulin are virtually the sole regulators of the energy-producing systems of the cells.

In a way I felt a sense of relief, for if I could now alter my approach a little to avoid his tender spots, I might be able to clear the matter up for both of us.

"You know, Dr. Cameron," I said carefully, "I think I'm doing a very poor job of communicating to you just what we're trying to accomplish in our research effort. Would you mind if I go back a bit and try to show you in a little more detail how we come to be using these tests at all?"

He nodded assent, but I felt he really had lost interest.

However, I made a brief sketch of the inception of our interest in mental illness, focusing on the discovery that some nutrients could apparently make some mentally ill persons more ill. I described how we had run hundreds of tests on individual vitamins and minerals in an effort to group together all of those nutrients that appeared to help a given type of patient, as well as to separate all of those nutrients that seemed to make this same type of patient more ill.

We referred to these alternative groupings simply as Type 1 and Type 2 formulas.

Having separated these materials more or less successfully, judging by how effective they were in helping mentally ill persons recover from illness, we were now faced by the urgent problem of finding some objective test that would tell us which formula, Type 1 or Type 2, would be more likely to benefit a given person.

So what we did was simple and direct. We ran before-and-after blood tests on a large number of items such as pH, CO_2 content, thyroid function, blood glucose, cholesterol, total lipids, urinary-steroids, blood electrolytes, and so on to see whether we could correlate an improvement or worsening in a patient's psychological condition while he was receiving either the Type 1 or thc Type 2 formula with some of the measures under study.

We found that of all the measures we tried, the plasma pH and the dissolved carbon dioxide and carbonic acid content of the blood were most closely related to the patient's psychological condition as well as to his reaction to the treatment he was receiving.

"For example," I said, "suppose this disturbed woman had actually been one of our research patients. We would have employed these tests and classified her as a 'Type 1 reactor.' And we could be fairly sure that this patient would probably respond favorably to our Type 1 grouping of vitamins and minerals."

Dr. Cameron's interest seemed to pick up. "If I recall correctly what you said earlier, you believed that her oxidation rate was slow, as you put it. Now, are you contending that your Type 1 formula acts to *increase* this rate?" he asked.

I told him that this was our hypothesis, based on both our observations and our general understanding of the biochemical likelihoods which might account for them.

"Now just suppose," Dr. Cameron asked, "that by some mix-up the patient is given the Type 2 formula, rather than the one you believe should be given. What then?"

I told him that the patient would become *more* psychologically disturbed, and the blood tests would show a *decrease,* rather than an increase, in the already very low level of dissolved carbon dioxide and carbonic acid.

Dr. Cameron looked at me thoughtfully. "I suppose you fully realize, Dr. Watson," he said, "that what you say you are doing is what everybody has always believed could never be done."

Throughout my discussions with Dr. Cameron I had never had the opportunity to mention some of the results we had obtained in our latest study. And although Dr. Cameron might not have known that it was indeed possible to increase or decrease the carbon dioxide in the blood by interfering with cellular enzymes by means of vitamins and minerals, I was pretty confident that the information I was about to show him might induce him to rethink the problem.

I pointed to a stack of charts on the desk in front of me. I picked up one labeled "Type 1–Slow Oxidizer—Type 2–Fast Oxidizer."

"Dr. Cameron," I said, "here are summaries of the results we have obtained in our latest study. I have just compiled them for publication.[1] One thing emerges from these data that–in my opinion–you can't either shake off or laugh off."

"Well, really! Whatever gave you the idea that one might do either?" Dr. Cameron asked.

"If you will look at just one set of comparative figures," I said. "Consider only the before-treatment values for dissolved carbon

[1] The data I showed Dr. Cameron are reproduced in the appendix at the end of the book.

dioxide and carbonic acid for the slow-oxidizing patients, as compared to what we call the fast oxidizers."

He glanced down the column, looking for the average values; they were 0.73 for the slow and 1.27 for the fast oxidizers.

There was really a whopping statistical difference between these values, and I wondered whether Dr. Cameron would be aware of just how big it was.

He was. He looked at me with that little smile, and said, "Well, at any rate, for *this* sample of patients, the difference between these types appears real enough."

I handed him another chart, which, if he could get the message at all, ought to jolt him a bit.

For the second chart showed that after treatment with the appropriate Type 1 or Type 2 formula of vitamins and minerals, there was no longer any significant difference between the slow-oxidizing and fast-oxidizing types of patients.

Finally he said reflectively, "I must say this appears to look good, really quite good. But obviously," he continued, his tone changing back to authority, "one needs much more evidence than what you have here. You know what I mean: not better evidence —to be sure—but more evidence, from other people."

I laughed something that wasn't a laugh.

"Do you think I've made a funny observation?" he asked.

"Well, in a sense," I replied. "What I was really thinking about was something you said a few minutes ago, and the incongruity it presents compared with what you have just said about the need for other scientists to take an interest in this line of research."

"And just what did I say that presents this incongruity?" he asked.

I repeated his words almost exactly. I said, "Well, here is what I believe you told me: 'I suppose you realize full well, Dr. Watson, that what you say you are doing is what everybody has always believed could never be done. And what's more, I'm pretty sure that you'll find the reaction I've had is very much the one you will meet practically everywhere in the scientific community.' "

In the preceding pages you may have found what is perhaps the best answer to Dr. Cameron's belief that "it can't be done"—the case histories of some of the actual people for whom it has been done, through research pointed in another direction–away from the futile conflicts of contending psychotherapies, toward the fundamental biological conditions that support all behavior.

Conclusion

If *serendipity* refers to the notion that discoveries of value may sometimes accidentally be made while one is searching for something quite different, then I suppose the true origin of the research reported in this book must be credited to serendipity.

While making observations on the sense of smell, seeking to determine what effect the ingestion of a biochemical such as thiamine chloride (vitamin B_1) had on the way that substance smelled, I first noticed what I imagined to be a rather definite change in mood following the intake of a large quantity–100 milligrams–of the biochemical being tested.

Subsequent testing confirmed this observation. Such changes in feelings appeared to be of two principal kinds: a brightening of spirits or a distinct depression of them. However, not always would such an effect follow and not always would the same chemical produce the same effect for the same person.

Although I did indeed discover that whether one can smell certain vitamins, as well as learn what they smell like, depends partly on the level of those substances in the system,[1] I soon became more interested in the notion that one's mood could be influenced –sometimes dramatically–by "mere" nutritional biochemicals.

[1] "The Effect of Thiamine on Thiamine Sniff Thresholds" (with Andrew L. Comrey and Elizabeth Klein), *Journal of General Psychology,* 1958, 69, 105–109.

I next spent several years trying to separate into groups the principal vitamins in terms of the simple criterion of whether or not each would elevate or depress the feelings of a subject under similar conditions. That is, if I found that thiamine would elevate one's mood at a given time, would, say, niacin also do so?

After I had achieved a quite tentative grouping of the vitamins into two groups, those in Group 1 appearing to have somewhat similar effects to one another while those in Group 2 had roughly the opposite effects, I decided to test them together as groups, instead of singly.

I was really unprepared for what happened, for it soon became clear that these combinations of nutritional biochemicals could, in a susceptible person—if the intake was large enough and continued long enough—produce symptoms that clinically resembled mental illness.

My next step was both obvious and necessary. If it were possible to experimentally induce what appeared to be something like neuroses and psychoses by biochemical means, and then again to reverse the process, might it not be likely that real mental illness had its roots in the biochemical malfunctioning of the nervous system?

At about this time the University of Minnesota studies in starvation came to my attention, in which were described mild as well as severe personality changes resulting from biochemical interference with the normal operation of the organism owing to reduced food intake. This research, together with my own observations, motivated me to ask Professor Andrew Comrey to join me in obtaining a research group of mentally ill subjects to explore the idea that mental illness was related to nutritional biochemical malfunctioning.

This first formal research study[2] confirmed two main points. The first was that some mental illness indeed resulted from nutritional biochemical malfunctioning, since it could be entirely relieved by biochemical means. The second was that treatment which might be appropriate for a given patient might be ineffective

[2] "Nutritional Replacement for Mental Illness" (with Andrew L. Comrey). *Journal of Psychology,* 1954, 38, 251–264.

or even harmful in another, even though both might appear to be afflicted with the "same" illness.

I spent the next ten years exploring the reasons for this finding, and some of the results of this research have been presented in the preceding chapters. Collaborating with me, and indeed making it possible for me to undertake and carry on this research, was W. D. Currier, M.D., who became medical director of the Lancaster Foundation for Scientific Research, which was organized to carry out this work.

The general research procedure was to run informal exploratory tests on individuals until specific points under study were elucidated. These were clinical tests of the reactions of mentally and emotionally upset patients to single vitamins and minerals as well as to various combinations of vitamins and minerals. In addition, we ran before-and-after-treatment blood and urine tests on these patients, to try to discover connections between the type of treatment and changes in blood and urine composition. The list of all the blood and urine tests we performed is quite lengthy, and is of insufficient general interest to be repeated here. It should be noted, however, that in all these tests we observed that the following variables were affected by the complex of vitamins and minerals being administered: blood glucose, total plasma lipids, cholesterol, plasma pH and related bicarbonate/carbonic acid ratio, urinary pH, salivary pH, blood pressure, and pulse.

After completing exploratory tests, we would then attempt to confirm our findings in a formal research group under experimental controls.

It should be mentioned that tests such as we were using are not tests to detect or to characterize mental illness. I know of none; and the research we have done seems to me to dim considerably the likelihood that such tests are possible in principle. We have found functional mental illness to be a reflection of disordered metabolism, principally involving the malfunctioning of enzyme systems. Consequently, blood tests that may be of use will likely be those that reflect the functioning of the enzymes, or those that detect factors that influence such functioning.

In particular, however, my main goal at this period was to discover some biochemical differences between the two groups of research patients who, although apparently suffering from the "same" type of mental illness—such as anxiety neurosis—yet responded oppositely to the identical treatment. We referred to these patients simply as Type 1 or Type 2 reactors. We did indeed find metabolic differences between them, which are discussed in detail in this book. The biochemical test that we found best discriminates between these two groups of patients is the carbonic acid level of the blood (actually the dissolved carbon dioxide plus carbonic acid), which intimately reflects the manner in which the tissues of the body are consuming fuel and creating energy. While a normal healthy adult will show a concentration of 1.35 mM/l of carbonic acid and dissolved carbon dioxide, what we have called slow oxidizers (Type 1) will have an average concentration of about one-half this much—0.73 mM/l, while fast oxidizers (Type 2) will have an average concentration of about 1.27 mM/l (see appendix). In addition to the free carbon dioxide level, there are other measures that may be useful, perhaps the best of which is the glucose tolerance test mentioned earlier.

More than 300 research subjects were involved in this work, some of whom were under study for five years or more. Most of these subjects were involved in casual exploratory tests, while of the total somewhat fewer than half participated in controlled studies that were published, each of which yielded statistically significant improvement rates.[3] In addition to patients involved directly in research, the tests developed and the treatment regimens have since been used by a number of physicians in clinical practice on large numbers of patients suffering from functional metabolic disorders.

Although the rate of improvement we have found among those

[3] "Differences in Intermediary Metabolism in Mental Illness," Monograph 2-V17, 1965, *Psychology Reports* (reprinted as the Appendix of this book); "Intensive Vitamin Therapy in Mental Illness" (with W. D. Currier), *Journal of Psychology,* 1959, 49, 67–81; "Vitamin Deficiencies in Mental Illness," *Journal of Psychology,* 1957, 43, 47–63; "Is Mental Illness Mental?" *Journal of Psychology,* 1956, 41, 323–343; "Nutritional Replacement for Mental Illness," *Journal of Psychology,* 1954, 38, 251–264.

suffering from virtually every kind of mental illness is very high—about 80 per cent—and we have seen dramatic case histories of complete clinical remissions in what heretofore have been considered almost intractable illness, still, in every experiment there has remained a small but resistant core of patients who have had either minimal improvement or none at all. Most often these patients also had previously been treated unsuccessfully by a wide variety of methods, including electroshock, drugs, and "analysis," suggesting the possibility that their difficulties were genetic in origin.

The fact that there are minimal improvements and outright failures in treating disturbed behavior psychochemically should occasion no surprise. This is indeed what one would expect if mental illness is a reflection of disordered metabolism, as I have suggested that it is. The human organism is of almost forbidding complexity when considered from the biochemical—which includes genetic—point of view. There are consequently an untold number of things that can and do go wrong—with genes, with hormones, with enzymes, with nutrition, with infection, with stress, with toxemia, and with structure. Although some of these factors have been discussed here, it clearly will take more time and research before the roles of all such possible etiological factors in mental illness are explored.

While the work reported in this book is research in a hopeful new direction, it is hardly more than a probing step toward understanding the foundations of disturbed behavior. The mentally and emotionally troubled person is one who isn't adequately accounted for by the prevailing medical yardsticks used to measure normal health. Unfailingly, our research patients had been judged by their physicians to be physically healthy when in fact they were not. In many cases the range of what is said to be "normal" on standard tests used in medicine is so large that a condition which seriously requires correction may be accepted as normal or borderline normal, and thus thought to have little significance. For example, the range of blood-sugar levels said to be normal is from 65 to 105 (mg./100 ml., venous blood, true glucose). For some people a blood-sugar level of 65 means psychochemical behavior, such as severe anxiety or depression. Such a person is ill and needs attention; yet the doctor can find nothing wrong. At the other end of the scale, a blood-sugar level of 105 may be one of the reasons a slow oxidizer is suicidally depressed. The depression lifts "miraculously" when the blood sugar is reduced–when his oxidation rate is increased–through nutritional treatment to 90. This person's initial blood-sugar level was an index of illness, yet the doctor failed to recognize it as such, for he had thought it to be "within normal range," or "high normal," and thus not important.

Let us consider still another example, somewhat similar but with a more obvious illogical twist: a schizophrenic girl whom we found to have a blood plasma pH of 7.35. The pH is a measure of the hydrogen ion concentration, which is an important variable affecting the rate of cellular energy production. When I mentioned to her doctor that we had found the pH to be 7.35, he said–and this is the standard, typical response–"Well, normal people have a pH of 7.35; *therefore* she is normal." Now just because normal people may in fact have a pH of 7.35 is insufficient reason for concluding that *all* people who have a pH of 7.35 are normal. For under nutritional biochemical treatment, when this girl recovered from her illness her plasma pH was found to be 7.45. Clearly the initial reading of 7.35 was *not* normal for her–it was an indicator of her illness, and her doctor failed to recognize it as such.

These examples point explicitly to the pressing need in research with the emotionally and mentally disturbed: to develop metabolic profiles that are characteristic of disturbed individuals *as such,* without reference to the norms established for the healthy and undisturbed. The very lack of such information is one of the principal reasons why physicians and medical researchers claim they can find "no physical causes for emotionally disturbed behavior," for the criteria they are employing as a basis for judging are simply not applicable. What is "normal" for a normal person is not necessarily "normal" for an emotionally disturbed person; he is in fact a different kind of person. These researchers are looking right at the evidences of physical abnormality they are seeking, while at once saying they can't find any.

Another urgent necessity in the research and treatment of disturbed behavior is to *stop* classifying patients solely in terms of psychological symptoms. Virtually all current and past research into disturbed behavior is vitiated by using psychological criteria as the only basis on which to classify patients for study. For example, two patients, both presenting symptoms of severe anxiety, may exhibit anxiety because of exactly opposite biochemical reasons. One may be burning sugar far too rapidly, the other far too slowly. Fast oxidizers must be distinguished from slow ones–and both from suboxidizers–if treatment is to succeed. Words such as *schizophrenia, manic-depression,* and *anxiety neurosis* tell us nothing whatever about the physical state of the individual, and in fact may mislead one into thinking that *all* schizophrenics, *all* manic-depressives, or *all* anxious patients are biochemically similar.

In addition to classifying patients in terms of types of metabolic disturbances in nutritional metabolism, as has been done in this book, much research is needed for discovering and describing other basic types of physical dysfunction, such as hormonal and genetic.

These general comments on the state of research in mental and emotional disturbances should again remind the reader of the really primitive level of our knowledge in this area, and of the attendant difficulty of securing effective help should it be required. The psychochemical and personality quizzes included earlier should be understood as being illustrative and suggestive rather than diagnostic. They alone should not be used as a basis for self-treatment, which under any circumstance is hazardous, but rather as a guide for seeking treatment.

Should you or anyone else need help it is advisable to go to your own physician, who can run the necessary tests and prescribe and supervise the proper treatment. In addition, your doctor, or a telephone call to the local medical society, will provide you with the names of physicians in general psychiatry who are oriented to look at one's problems from the physical–rather than from the mere psychological–point of view.

While the hoped-for goal of this book is to stimulate interest, research, and treatment in a relatively uncharted direction, it is also the author's hope that it will help those who read it to better understand the origins of their difficulties, and also to help them obtain effective treatment.

Appendix

DIFFERENCES IN INTERMEDIARY METABOLISM IN MENTAL ILLNESS

George Watson
Lancaster Foundation for Scientific Research

Summary.—Exploratory tests of the hypothesis that enzymatic blocks due to unsuspected co-factor deficiencies might be a causal factor in functional mental illness revealed that treatment with certain vitamins or minerals in some instances could apparently make mentally ill *S*s more ill. Extensive clinical tests led to separation of the principal vitamins and minerals into groups in terms of whether or not they would improve or worsen the condition of a given *S*. Two basic types of mentally ill *S*s, Types I and II, and two corresponding types of vitamins and minerals were tentatively established. Blood studies revealed statistically significant differences between *S*s classified as Type I or as Type II, the greatest differences being found in the plasma pH and in the dissolved $CO_2 + H_2CO_3$. Preliminary exploration of the effect of treatment indicates these variables co-vary with psychological status of *S* when given appropriate vitamins and minerals. Since Type I *S*s showed an *increase* in dissolved $CO_2 + H_2CO_3$ with treatment, it is suggested that they are *slow oxidizers,* and Type II *S*s who show a *decrease* are *fast oxidizers.*

Several types of anomalies involving intermediary metabolism have been reported in schizophrenics, including nitrogen retention in periodic catatonia, ketonuria, abnormal glucose tolerance, as well as others (9). These findings, although not characteristic of schizophrenia in general, nevertheless suggest that in some mentally ill patients biochemical lesions may exist in the mechanisms for energy release from nutrients, since nitrogen retention, ketonuria, and abnormal glucose tolerance reflect abnormalities in protein, fat, and carbohydrate metabolism.

This possibility appears to gain support from the discovery that mental illness may be induced in emotionally healthy volunteer *S*s when they are placed on an experimental semi-starvation diet (7). Although mental illness induced in this manner probably does not result from a metabolic defect, but rather from a caloric deficit, the end-result may be the same, namely, an insufficient production of energy resulting in impaired functioning of the central and peripheral nervous systems.

The report that starvation-induced neuroses and psychoses cannot be differentiated clinically from "functional" mental illness—which many believe to originate in psychological conflict and trauma—is particularly striking (1).

It has long been known that a deficiency of a single vitamin, nicotinic acid, can cause psychosis, and that this illness can be cured by administering niacin or its amide. Other vitamins in addition to niacin also have been implicated in the etiology of specific mental disorders (8). Since several of the vitamins and some of the trace minerals function as coenzymes or as constituents of enzymes in both the Embden-Meyerhoff (glycolytic) and Kreb's (tricarboxylic acid) metabolic pathways, if mental illness can result from malfunctioning of such energy producing systems, it appears that the deficiency of one or more vitamins and/or minerals could play either a primary or secondary role in the etiology of some neuroses and psychoses.

Experiments designed to explore the hypothesis that enzymatic blocks due to unsuspected co-factor deficiencies might be a causal factor in functional mental illness produced an altogether surprising result, namely, that treatment with vitamins and minerals in many instances could apparently make mentally ill patients more ill (11). For example, it was frequently found that two *S*s, paired as closely as possible for age, sex, duration of illness, clinical symptoms, and psychological test scores, would respond differently to an identical combination of vitamins and minerals, one improving markedly with the other becoming much more ill. In the latter case, discontinuing the treatment generally resulted in improvement within a few days.

Consequently, it appears that certain vitamins and minerals may benefit some mentally ill *S*s but seem to worsen the condition of others with similar symptoms. This finding led to trial-by-error clinical tests to determine whether it would be possible to separate the principal vitamins and minerals into groups in terms of the criterion of whether or not they would worsen or improve a major symptom such as anxiety, depression, or paranoid reaction in a given *S*. For example, an *S* whose dominant symptom was anxiety was instructed to take a tablet of thiamine chloride (100 mg.) both during an attack of panic and when he felt relatively secure. Trials such as this with thiamine showed that in some *S*s noticeable relief from anxiety apparently was afforded during an attack and that periods of anxiety apparently became more widely separated. On the other hand, thiamine seemed to produce the opposite result in other *S*s presenting a similar clinical picture of anxiety neurosis. Since clinical trials such as this with thiamine were alternated with placebos without *S*'s knowledge, it appears that vitamin B_1, for example, can worsen the symptoms of anxiety in some *S*s as well as bring relief to others.

Extensive exploratory trials of this kind with the principal vitamins and minerals were performed over a period of several years, utilizing over 200 mentally ill *S*s who exhibited a very wide range of psychological disorders. This research resulted in the tentative establishment of two basic types of mentally ill *S*s and two basic classes of vitamins and minerals (Table 1). *S*s were designated as "Type I" if they appeared to respond favorably to "Type I" vitamins and/or minerals and unfavorably to "Type II" vitamins and/or minerals. *S*s were designated as "Type II" if they appeared to respond favorably to "Type II" vitamins and/or minerals and unfavorably to "Type I" vitamins and/or minerals.

Blood studies showed large and significant statistical differences between patients who were retrospectively classified as Type I ($N = 12$) or Type II ($N = 12$) in terms of the success of treatment with the corresponding Type I or Type II vitamins and minerals. Table 2 summarizes the before-treatment values for venous plasma pH, dissolved carbon dioxide plus carbonic acid, total lipids, and fasting blood sugar in 24 *S*s, 12 in each group, showing significant differences between the group means for pH, $CO_2 + H_2CO_3$, and lipids, while the blood sugar difference is not quite significant at the 5% level.

These particular tests proved to be the most promising of many that were investigated for their possible relationship to the Type I-Type II classification of *S*s. Since the greatest differences between the two types of *S*s were found in the plasma pH and dissolved carbon dioxide, a small pilot experiment was undertaken to explore the hypothesis

TABLE 1

PRINCIPAL VITAMINS AND MINERALS CLASSIFIED IN TERMS OF FAVORABLE/UNFAVORABLE RESPONSE CRITERION IN TYPES I AND II MENTALLY ILL *Ss*

Type I	Type II
Vitamin D	Vitamin A
Vitamin K	Vitamin E
Ascorbic Acid	Vitamin B_{12}
Biotin	Nicotinamide
Folic Acid	Pantothenic Acid
Pyridoxine	Choline*
PABA	Inositol*
Niacin	Citrus Bioflavonoid Complex*
Riboflavin	
Thiamine	
Iron	Calcium
Potassium	Iodine
Magnesium	Phosphorous
Copper	Sodium
Chloride	Zinc
Manganese	

*This substance is arbitrarily classified as a "vitamin" for the purposes of this discussion.

that these variables were related both to the Type I-Type II classifications as well as to the psychological conditions of the mentally ill *S*s so classified, and that they covaried with the changing psychological status of *S*s under treatment.

THE EXPERIMENT

Twenty unhospitalized ambulatory *S*s were selected for an 8-mo. study on the basis of the severity of their illnesses and the length of time they had been ill. Every *S* had an extended history of mental illness for which he previously had been treated without significant success. Twelve had received electroshock therapy, 18 had been under psychotherapy, and all had received one or more forms of psychotropic drugs. Eleven of the 20 were diagnosed by a psychiatrist as psychotic (schizophrenic), while 9 had been diagnosed as neurotic (anxiety, depressive, obsessive-compulsive).[1]

Brief psychological case histories were recorded in an initial inter-

[1] Detailed case histories of the individuals who participated in this study will be published elsewhere.

TABLE 2

DIFFERENCES IN VENOUS PLASMA PH, DISSOLVED CO_2 + H_2CO_3, TOTAL LIPIDS, AND FASTING BLOOD SUGAR BETWEEN TYPE I ($N = 12$) AND TYPE II ($N = 12$) MENTALLY ILL *S*s

S	Venous Plasma pH		Dissolved CO_2 + H_2CO_3 (mM/1)		Total Lipids		Blood Sugar	
	Type I	Type II	Type I	Type II	Type I	Type II	Type I	Type II
1	7.48	7.37	1.02	1.26	880	1315	56	93
2	7.51	7.39	.97	1.23	1150	930	76	59
3	7.51	7.45	.99	1.11	1180	1125	90	105
4	7.55	7.39	.74	1.23	830	1125	86	80
5	7.55	7.42	.74	1.05	500	880	94	53
6	7.50	7.39	.69	1.20	550	1345	108	80
7	7.56	7.36	1.02	1.29	725	1235	122	76
8	7.50	7.45	.91	1.09	665	1035	104	70
9	7.52	7.40	.93	1.22	638	1095	83	96
10	7.53	7.40	.90	1.22	325	1025	76	48
11	7.47	7.39	1.06	1.18	590	685	84	86
12	7.51	7.43	.87	1.09	590	665	108	56
M	7.52	7.40	.91	1.18	719	1038	91	75
	$t = 9.73$*		$t = 6.65$		$t = 3.30$		$t = 1.97$	

*$t_{.05} = 2.074$; $t_{.01} = 2.819$.

view, together with dietary information in order to determine approximate protein, fat, and carbohydrate intakes. All *S*s reported that they were eating mixed diets which generally represented the basic food groups. In addition to dietary data, medical histories were also obtained, and routine physical examinations with laboratory tests were given to all *S*s. The venous plasma pH and the CO_2 content were determined both at the beginning and at the end of the experiment.

The psychological progress of each *S* was checked by the author clinically in a monthly 30-min. interview, at which time adjustments in medication were made if necessary. *S*s were classified as Type I ($N = 10$) if their initial pH was 7.47 or higher, and as Type II ($N = 10$) if their initial pH was 7.45 or lower. These limits were selected on the basis of previous research (Table 2) and represent the lowest pH measured in a Type I *S*, as well as the highest pH determined for a Type II *S*. Before-treatment test values for the two groups are presented in Table 3. The differences between mean values for the Type I and Type II *S*s were statistically significant for all 3 biochemical measures (see Table 3).

The formulas administered to each of the two types of *S*s are listed in Table 4. Type I *S*s were given the formula of Type I vitamins and

TABLE 3

BEFORE-TREATMENT DIFFERENCES IN VENOUS PLASMA pH, BICARBONATE, AND DISSOLVED $CO_2 + H_2CO_3$ BETWEEN TYPE I ($N = 10$) AND TYPE II ($N = 10$) MENTALLY ILL *S*s

S	Venous Plasma pH		Plasma Bicarbonate		Dissolved $CO_2+H_2CO_3$	
	Type I	Type II	Type I	Type II	Type I	Type II
1	7.55	7.35	13.50	23.50	.48	1.32
2	7.50	7.36	18.50	23.50	.73	1.29
3	7.55	7.38	22.50	24.00	.79	1.25
4	7.55	7.36	17.00	23.50	.60	1.29
5	7.56	7.40	26.00	24.00	.90	1.20
6	7.50	7.35	17.50	22.50	.69	1.26
7	7.55	7.37	18.50	23.50	.65	1.25
8	7.49	7.33	24.00	23.00	.97	1.35
9	7.55	7.36	21.00	22.50	.74	1.23
10	7.56	7.35	20.50	23.50	.71	1.32
M	7.54	7.36	19.90	23.35	.73	1.27
	$t = 5.22$*		$t = 2.94$		$t = 11.75$	

*$t_{.05} = 2.101$. $t_{.01} = 2.878$.

TABLE 4

VITAMIN-MINERAL COMBINATIONS USED IN EXPERIMENTAL TREATMENT OF TYPES I AND II MENTALLY ILL *S*s*

Type I Formula		Type II Formula	
Vitamin B_1	10 mg.	Vitamin A	25,000 IU
Vitamin B_2	10 mg.	Vitamin E	100 IU
Vitamin B_6	10 mg.	Vitamin B_{12}	10 mcg.
PABA	25 mg.	Nicotinamide	200 mg.
Niacin	25 mg.	Pantothenate	50 mg.
Ascorbic Acid	300 mg.	Choline	300 mg.
Vitamin D	2500 IU	Inositol	90 mg.
Potassium Citrate	900 mg.	Bioflavonoids	350 mg.
Magnesium Chloride	100 mg.	Calcium	330 mg.
Copper Gluconate	.6 mg.	Phosphorous	250 mg.
Manganese Oxide	10 mg.	Iodine	.45 mg.
		Zinc Sulfate	10 mg.

*The quantities listed for each type formula represent the basic dosage, which was administered in capsule form, three times daily, after meals. Individual variations in response to treatment occurred, most frequently requiring a reduction in the number of times daily the basic dosage was given.

minerals and Type II *S*s were given the formula of Type II vitamins and minerals.

Results

*S*s were evaluated clinically by the author and placed in one of three categories: (i) clinical remission of symptoms, (ii) marked reduction in intensity of symptoms, or (iii) noticeable reduction in intensity of symptoms.[2]

An *S* was judged to have achieved a clinical remission of symptoms if the major symptoms for which he was being treated were no longer evident. For example, when an obsessive-compulsive neurotic who was a compulsive eater no longer thought about food and no longer consumed huge quantities, she was considered to have shown a clinical remission of symptoms.

An *S* was judged to have achieved a marked reduction in intensity of symptoms if improvement occurred to the point where the manifestations of illness no longer constituted a major problem for him. For example, an *S* was considered as having shown a marked reduction in intensity of symptoms who at the start of treatment presented a severe anxiety neurosis which prevented his driving a car and working, while at the end of the experiment he had obtained a job and drove regularly, although he was still anxiety-prone under stress.

Finally, an *S* was judged to have achieved a noticeable reduction in intensity of symptoms when definite behavioral changes occurred although the illness was still clearly manifest. For example, a withdrawn schizophrenic *S* was judged as showing a noticeable reduction in intensity of symptoms when at the start of treatment he would rarely speak to anyone but his mother and would not voluntarily leave the house, but just prior to the end of the experimental period he had voluntarily taken a trip of several days' duration with members of a radio listeners' club he had joined, after which, however, he exhibited his previous pattern of withdrawal.

Evaluated in the manner just described, every *S* in the experiment showed psychological improvement: 11 out of 20 (55%) were classified as showing clinical remission of symptoms, 5 out of 20 (25%) were classified as showing marked reduction in intensity of symptoms, while 4 out of 20 (20%) were classified as showing noticeable reduction in intensity of symptoms (Table 5).

These psychological improvements were accompanied by changes in

[2] Although previous studies (10, 12, 13) employed both clinical evaluations made by the present author as well as the Minnesota Multiphasic Personality Inventory, the latter was not used in the present experiment since some *S*s were too disturbed to be evaluated in this manner. However, in all of the previous studies where both clinical judgment by the author and MMPI were used together, each type of evaluation yielded similar confidence levels in assessing psychological change. It should be remarked that in none of the previous experiments was a significant placebo response recorded.

TABLE 5

CLINICAL IMPROVEMENTS IN TYPES I AND II MENTALLY ILL *S*s

Type I					Type II				
S	Age (yr.)	Sex	Diagnosis	Evaluation*	*S*	Age	Sex	Diagnosis	Evaluation*
1	43	M	Depressive Reaction	+++	1	53	F	Schizophrenic Reaction	+
2	54	F	Schizophrenic Reaction	+++	2	62	F	Schizophrenic Reaction	+++
3	48	F	Schizophrenic Reaction	+++	3	29	F	Anxiety Neurosis	++
4	55	F	Schizophrenic Reaction	+++	4	51	M	Anxiety Neurosis	++
5	27	F	Schizophrenic Reaction	++	5	21	F	Obsessive-Compulsive	+++
6	49	F	Schizophrenic Reaction	++−	6	28	F	Obsessive-Compulsive	+
7	56	F	Anxiety Neurosis	+	7	24	M	Depressive Reaction	+++
8	32	M	Schizophrenic Reaction	++	8	43	M	Schizophrenic Reaction	+++
9	22	F	Anxiety Neurosis	++	9	29	M	Schizophrenic Reaction	+++
10	24	M	Schizophrenic Reaction	+++	10	39	M	Anxiety Neurosis	+

*+++ = Clinical remission of symptoms.
++ = Marked reduction in intensity of symptoms.
+ = Noticeable reduction in intensity of symptoms.

the biochemical variables under study, the initial differences in plasma pH, plasma bicarbonate, and dissolved carbon dioxide plus carbonic acid between Type I and Type II *S*s disappearing with treatment.

At the start of the experiment the average plasma pH of Type I *S*s was 7.54, while at the end of the experiment it was 7.43 (Table 6).

TABLE 6

BEFORE AND AFTER TREATMENT DIFFERENCES IN VENOUS PLASMA pH, BICARBONATE, AND DISSOLVED $CO_2 + H_2CO_3$ IN TYPE I MENTALLY ILL *S*s ($N = 10$)

S No. and Sex	Age (yr.)	Plasma pH		Bicarbonate (mM/l)		Dissolved $CO_2 + H_2CO_3$ (mM/l)	
		Before	After	Before	After	Before	After
1 M	43†	7.55	7.41	13.50	23.50	.48	1.14
2 F	54‡	7.50	7.44	18.50	24.00	.73	1.09
3 F	48‡	7.55	7.45	22.50	22.00	.79	.98
4 F	55‡	7.55	7.42	17.00	24.00	.60	1.14
5 F	27‡	7.56	7.45	26.00	27.50	.90	1.22
6 F	49‡	7.50	7.43	17.50	24.50	.69	1.14
7 F	56§	7.55	.7.46	18.50	22.00	.65	.96
8 M	32‡	7.49	7.42	24.00	25.50	.97	1.22
9 F	22§	7.55	·7.42	21.00	20.05	.74	.97
10 M	24‡	7.56	7.42	20.50	24.50	.71	1.17
M		7.54	7.43	19.90	23.80	.73	1.10
		$t = 10.74$*		$t = 3.46$		$t = 8.01$	

*$t_{.05} = 2.262$; $t_{.01} = 3.250$.
Note.—Diagnosis: †Depressive Reaction; ‡Schizophrenic Reaction; §Anxiety Neurosis.

Type II *S*s had an average plasma pH of 7.36 before treatment, while after treatment it was 7.46 (Table 7). Thus the initial mean pH values for Type I and Type II *S*s of 7.54 and 7.36, respectively, were no longer present after treatment, at which time the values for each group were 7.43 and 7.46, respectively. These changes in pH for each type of *S* are statistically significant well beyond the 1% level of confidence, using the *t* test.

The beginning values for plasma bicarbonate in Type I *S*s averaged 19.90 millimoles per liter (mM/l) as compared to 23.80 mM/l at the end of the treatment period. Type II *S*s had an average initial plasma bicarbonate level of 23.35 mM/l and an after treatment level of 24.15 mM/l. Thus the before treatment differences in this variable between Type I and Type II *S*s of 19.90 mM/l and 23.35 mM/l, respectively, were not present at the end of the experiment, when the bicarbonate levels for the two types of *S*s were 23.80 mM/l and 24.15 mM/l, respectively.

TABLE 7

BEFORE AND AFTER TREATMENT DIFFERENCES IN VENOUS PLASMA PH, BICARBONATE, AND DISSOLVED $CO_2 + H_2CO_3$ IN TYPE II MENTALLY ILL *S*s ($N = 10$)

S No. and Sex	Age (yr.)	Plasma pH Before	Plasma pH After	Bicarbonate (mM/l) Before	Bicarbonate (mM/l) After	Dissolved $CO_2 + H_2CO_3$ (mM/l) Before	Dissolved $CO_2 + H_2CO_3$ (mM/l) After
1 F	53‡	7.35	7.47	23.50	23.50	1.32	1.00
2 F	62‡	7.36	7.42	23.50	23.50	1.29	1.12
3 F	29§	7.38	7.47	24.00	26.00	1.25	1.10
4 M	51§	7.36	7.45	23.50	24.50	1.29	1.10
5 F	21Ş	7.40	7.45	24.00	25.50	1.20	1.13
6 F	28Ş	7.35	7.45	22.50	25.00	1.26	1.11
7 M	24†	7.37	7.51	23.50	24.50	1.25	.95
8 M	43‡	7.33	7.50	23.00	23.50	1.35	.93
9 M	29‡	7.36	7.42	22.50	22.00	1.23	1.05
10 M	39§	7.35	7.47	23.50	23.50	1.32	1.00
M		7.36	7.46	23.35	24.15	1.27	1.04
		$t = 8.26$*		$t = 2.59$		$t = 6.70$	

*$t_{.05} = 2.262$; $t_{.01} = 3.250$.
Note.—Diagnosis: †Depressive Reaction; ‡Schizophrenic Reaction; §Anxiety Neurosis; ŞObsessive Compulsive Neurosis.

Each type of *S* registered increases in plasma bicarbonate that were significant statistically (see Tables 6 and 7).

The initial concentration of dissolved carbon dioxide plus carbonic acid for Type I *S*s averaged .73 mM/l, which increased to 1.10 mM/l at the end of the experiment (see Table 6). Type II *S*s had an average initial level for this variable of 1.27 mM/l, which decreased to 1.04 mM/l at the end of the treatment period (see Table 7). Thus the beginning differences between the two types of *S*s for dissolved carbon dioxide plus carbonic acid, represented by values of .73 mM/l and 1.27 mM/l, respectively, were not present after treatment, when the levels for this variable were 1.10 mM/l and 1.04 mM/l, respectively. These changes for both Type I and Type II *S*s are statistically significant ($p < .01$).

Tables 6 and 7 summarize these before and after treatment values for plasma pH, bicarbonate, and dissolved carbon dioxide plus carbonic acid for Type I and Type II *S*s. In each case the *t* test for the differences between the correlated means was used.

DISCUSSION

Of particular interest from the viewpoint of intermediary metabolism is that at the beginning of the experiment the Type I *S*s had an average level of dissolved $CO_2 + H_2CO_3$ that was 43% less than that of Type

II *Ss* (.73 mM/l compared to 1.27 mM/l) ($p < .00001$). That this is apparently a real characteristic of Type I *Ss* rather than an artifact due to classificatory decision in experimental design is suggested by the fact that this difference disappeared with experimental treatment.

In order to discuss possible reasons for these observations, some elementary background information must be considered.

As carbon dioxide and water are the major end-products of the oxidation of all types of food, the amount of CO_2 that is produced by the tissues, as related to the amount of oxygen that is consumed, provides the principal basis for measuring the energy output of the organism.

Carbon dioxide enters the plasma as dissolved gas from tissue cells where it is formed by the processes of intermediary metabolism. In the extracellular fluid a small amount is hydrated to form carbonic acid:

$$CO_2 + H_2O \leftrightarrows H_2CO_3 \qquad [1]$$

Carbonic acid ionizes according to the equation:

$$H_2CO_3 \leftrightarrows H^+ + HCO_3^- \qquad [2]$$

The bicarbonate ion HCO_3^- is normally balanced by sodium. The hydrogen ion concentration of the extracellular fluid is determined by the degree of dissociation of H_2CO_3 and by the amount of available base. These relationships are summarized by the Henderson-Hasselbalch equation:

$$\text{pH} = 6.1 + \log \frac{[HCO_3^-]}{[H_2CO_3]} \qquad [3]$$

According to Equation [3], when the bicarbonate concentration is 27 mM/l and the concentration of dissolved carbon dioxide plus carbonic acid is 1.35 mM/l, the plasma pH will be 7.40. When this ratio is based upon a pH of 7.40, a bicarbonate level of 27 mM/l and a dissolved carbon dioxide plus carbonic acid level of 1.35 mM/l, it is considered to represent the theoretical "ideal normal" (3).

Although there are conflicting reports in the literature as to what constitute "normal" ranges for these variables for healthy adults, very close experimental confirmation of the theoretical normal values just cited has recently been obtained in a careful study (2).

Under conditions of normal pH, the volume of carbon dioxide produced divided by the volume of oxygen consumed in a given period allows the calculation of the respiratory quotient (R.Q.), which provides a clue to the type of food being oxidized. For example, the R.Q. of carbohydrate is 6/6 or 1, being oxidized according to the equation:

$$C_6H_{12}O_6 + 6O_2 = 6CO_2 + 6H_2O$$

The average respiratory quotients for fat and protein are 0.71 and 0.80, respectively, while an "average" mixed diet gives a R.Q. of about 0.85. Since the brain has a R.Q. of between 0.9 and 1.0, it depends mainly upon carbohydrate for energy. Approximately 90% of the brain's respiration can be accounted for by glucose consumption, even though it possesses both the anaerobic (glycolytic) and aerobic (citric acid) metabolic pathways, and appears to be capable of oxidizing the same substrates as do other tissues.

The volume of carbon dioxide expired during normal respiration is related to the partial pressure of CO_2 in the alveolar air. Since the blood volume of dissolved $CO_2 + H_2CO_3$ is in equilibrium with the pCO_2 of the alveolar air, the higher the blood level of dissolved CO_2 plus carbonic acid, the larger is the percentage of carbohydrate being oxidized. Conversely, in uncontrolled diabetes, for example, where fat and protein are oxidized instead of carbohydrate, the R.Q. may be 0.70, with a proportionate decrease in dissolved CO_2 level.

In addition to the types of food being oxidized, there are a great number of other conditions which can cause deviations in the volume of CO_2 being produced, as well as deviations in hydrogen ion and bicarbonate concentrations. Because of the considerable complexity of this problem, there consequently may be numerous possible reasons for the observed differences between Types I and II mentally ill *S*s other than the metabolic ones to be considered in what follows. The explanations advanced, however, appear to accord with the observations, whether or not they do account for them.

Possibly the major clue to understanding the results reported in this study lies in the fact that some mentally ill *S*s apparently can be made more ill by administration of certain vitamins and minerals. Since some of the substances which exert such adverse effects are implicated principally in fat and protein metabolism, while the nervous system depends principally upon the oxidation of carbohydrate, it appears that the manner in which fat and protein are utilized in general intermediary metabolism may exert an indirect effect upon brain respiration. This is known to happen, for example, in diabetes, where circulating blood ketones resulting from the excessive breakdown of fat may actually lower cerebral respiration to the point of coma.

A consideration of the most important metabolic roles played by several of the vitamins that produce untoward psychological reactions in some mentally ill persons suggests that two major types of disturbances in intermediary metabolism may be involved: (i) a differentially slow oxidation of carbohydrates and glucogenic amino acids, resulting in a slow but preferential utilization of fats and ketogenic amino acids, and (ii) a disproportionally fast oxidation of carbohydrates and glucogenic amino acids, together with a slower, but still more rapid than normal, oxidation of fats and ketogenic amino acids.

The Type I *S*s represent the "slow oxidizers," while the Type II *S*s represent the "fast oxidizers."

The following discussion of this hypothesis will only undertake to illustrate briefly the lines of reasoning involved, since a more complete analysis would require lengthy treatment.

Among the vitamins in the Type I grouping which appear to worsen the psychological symptoms of Type II "fast oxidizing" *S*s to the greatest degree are thiamine, niacin, pyridoxine, and riboflavin.

The pyrophosphoric ester of thiamine (TPP) participates in the major oxidative decarboxylations which lead to the formation of carbon dioxide. Probably the most important of these is the decarboxylation of pyruvic acid to acetylcoenzyme A, which can then in turn be oxidized in the tricarboxylic acid cycle to CO_2 and H_2O. In addition to thiamine, niacin as nicotinamide adenine dinucleotide (NAD) also participates in this reaction. The absence of thiamine is known to prevent the breakdown of pyruvate, resulting in incomplete carbohydrate oxidation and in the accumulation of both pyruvate and lactate in the blood.

On the other hand, the administration of relatively large amounts of thiamine or niacin may possibly result in an increase in the rate of decarboxylation of pyruvate to acetylcoenzyme A. If this were to occur in the presence of sufficient amounts of substrate as well as of all of the other co-factors necessary to the operation of the Kreb's cycle at an increased rate, the result would be an increase in the volume of carbon dioxide entering the blood from the tissues.

Pyridoxine (as pyridoxal phosphate), as well as riboflavin (as flavin adenine dinucleotide, FAD), play prominent roles in the catabolism of amino acids. Pyridoxal phosphate is required as a prosthetic group in transamination, as well as functioning as coenzyme in the alternate pathway of amino acid breakdown of decarboxylation. FAD participates in the oxidation deamination of amino acids.

Both the transamination and deamination of amino acids yield keto acids, some of which (such as pyruvic, oxaloacetic, and α-oxoglutaric) are formed from glucogenic amino acids and are oxidized in the same manner as are carbohydrates.

Since pyridoxine and riboflavin are essential to the catabolism of amino acids, some of which are ultimately oxidized in the same metabolic pathways as are carbohydrates, it appears possible that under appropriate conditions excess amounts of either vitamin could accelerate the rate of operation of the tricarboxylic acid cycle by increasing the rate of formation of pyruvic, oxaloacetic, and α-oxoglutaric acids.

On the hypothesis that Type II *S*s are "fast oxidizers," differing from Type I "slow oxidizers" principally in that they oxidize carbohydrate and glucogenic amino acids at a more rapid rate than do the latter, the administration of vitamins and minerals that play an important role in their breakdown might be expected to result in a further increase in the rate at which such "fast oxidizing" *S*s produce carbon dioxide. Such an increased volume of CO_2 would also be expected to elevate disproportionally the dissolved $CO_2 + H_2CO_3$ blood level, since hypothetically it would reflect the increased oxidation of carbohydrate and glucogenic amino acids.

This interpretation of the reason why thiamine, niacin, and other Type I vitamins and minerals aggravate the conditions of Type II *S*s is suggested by blood tests from five such "fast oxidizing" *S*s whose psychological conditions were inadvertently worsened when they were administered Type I vitamins and minerals while undergoing experimental treatment (Table 8).[3] These show decreases in plasma pH with disproportional increases in dissolved carbon dioxide plus carbonic

TABLE 8

BEFORE AND AFTER TREATMENT DIFFERENCES IN VENOUS PLASMA PH, BICARBONATE, AND DISSOLVED $CO_2 + H_2CO_3$ IN TYPE II "FAST OXIDIZING" MENTALLY ILL *S*s WHOSE PSYCHOLOGICAL SYMPTOMS WERE AGGRAVATED BY INAPPROPRIATE THERAPY

S	Plasma pH		Bicarbonate (mM/l)		Dissolved $CO_2 + H_2CO_3$ (mM/l)	
	Before	After	Before	After	Before	After
1	7.42	7.39	25.50	23.50	1.22	1.20
2	7.38	7.35	23.00	23.50	1.20	1.32
3	7.45	7.42	21.00	20.50	.93	.98
4	7.44	7.38	28.50	24.00	1.30	1.25
5	7.45	7.35	20.00	22.50	.89	1.26
M	7.43	7.38	23.60	22.80	1.10	1.20
	$t = 3.63, .05 > p > .01$		$t = 0.68$, n.s.		$t = 1.25$, n.s.	

[3] Data on these 5 *S*s were obtained in exploratory tests which preceded the experiment reported in this paper.

acid. The direction of these changes is the opposite of those that occur when psychological improvement is obtained with appropriate therapy and are what would be expected by the hypothesis under consideration.

In contrast to the "fast oxidizing" Type II mentally ill *S*s just considered, Type I *S*s appear to be "slow oxidizers" whose poor utilization of carbohydrate and glucogenic amino acids results in a slow but preferential utilization of fats and ketogenic amino acids. On this hypothesis it would be expected that the intake of vitamins that might tend to favor the increased oxidation of fats and ketogenic amino acids when carbohydrate metabolism is depressed would also tend to worsen the psychological conditions of such *S*s, principally because the normal oxidation of fatty acids depends upon the breakdown of carbohydrates.

The first step in the oxidation of fatty acids requires their activation to acetylcoenzyme A, utilizing adenosine triphosphate (ATP) as a source of energy. Since ATP is principally formed as the result of the final stages of carbohydrate metabolism, if this is not proceeding normally, fat oxidation is also reduced.

However, assuming that sufficient ATP is available from glycolysis, the acetyl-coA formed in the initial phase of fatty acid oxidation condenses with oxaloacetic acid to form citrate, which is subsequently oxidized to carbon dioxide and water in the Kreb's cycle. When carbohydrate metabolism is faulty there will not be enough oxaloacetic acid to combine with the acetyl-coA being formed. As a consequence, acetoacetic acid is produced, some of which is decarboxylated to acetone, while some is reduced to β-hydroxybutyric acid. Acetoacetic acid, β-hydroxybutyric acid, and acetone are ketone bodies which if formed may be oxidized to CO_2 and H_2O through the citric acid cycle in extrahepatic tissue. Here again, however, it is requisite that carbohydrate oxidation is proceeding normally, otherwise ketone bodies will accumulate in the blood and appear in the urine.

Under the conditions outlined above it is evident that any factor which might tend to increase the oxidation of fatty acids will further increase the need for the efficient oxidation of carbohydrates. With this relationship in view, the question of why Type I "slow oxidizing" *S*s appear to be made more ill by certain vitamins may be considered.

Two of the nutrients in the Type II grouping for which some of the metabolic functions are known and which appear to worsen the psychological conditions of most Type I *S*s are choline and pantothenate.

Choline is used by the body in the synthesis of phospholipids, which are one of the three principal lipid components of the plasma. Since the ingestion of phospholipid causes marked and persistent hyperlipemia

(14), the intake of excessive amounts of choline may elevate plasma lipid levels, since this substance is known to stimulate the rate of choline phospholipid synthesis. Elevated lipid levels increase the need for carbohydrate metabolites and in their absence may produce ketosis (14).

Pantothenic acid is a constituent of coenzyme A, which, together with a specific protein apoenzyme, functions in several reversible acetylation reactions in fat, protein, and carbohydrate metabolism. As noted above, the first step in the oxidation of fatty acids is their condensation with coenzyme A to form acetyl-coA, which, under conditions of normal carbohydrate metabolism, condenses with oxaloacetic acid to form citric acid. When carbohydrate oxidation is depressed, however, the acetyl-coA may accumulate faster than it can be utilized, resulting in the formation of ketone bodies. This state of affairs might possibly be aggravated if the intake of excessive amounts of pantothenate resulted in the formation of added coenzyme A, which could then in turn participate in the initial phase of fatty acid oxidation, consequently increasing the need for ATP and oxaloacetic acid.

On the hypothesis that the principal reason why Type I *S*s have disproportionately low average plasma levels of dissolved $CO_2 + H_2CO_3$ is that their carbohydrate metabolism is depressed, it would be anticipated that the administration of vitamins and minerals that might tend to increase fatty acid breakdown with the consequent increase in demands for carbohydrate metabolites such as oxaloacetic acid would also result in the further lowering of plasma levels of dissolved $CO_2 + H_2CO_3$, with a resulting increase in plasma pH.

Table 9 presents blood tests on 4 Type I *S*s whose psychological

TABLE 9

BEFORE AND AFTER TREATMENT DIFFERENCES IN VENOUS PLASMA PH, BICARBONATE, AND DISSOLVED $CO_2 + H_2CO_3$ IN TYPE I "SLOW OXIDIZING" MENTALLY ILL *S*S WHOSE PSYCHOLOGICAL SYMPTOMS WERE AGGRAVATED BY INAPPROPRIATE THERAPY

S	Plasma pH		Bicarbonate (mM/l)		Dissolved $CO_2 + H_2CO_3$ (mM/l)	
	Before	After	Before	After	Before	After
1	7.47	7.56	25.00	26.00	1.14	.90
2	7.45	7.49	19.00	24.00	.84	.97
3	7.50	7.55	22.00	19.00	.87	.67
4	7.46	7.52	24.50	22.00	1.06	.83
M	7.47	7.52	22.62	22.75	.98	.84
	$t = 6.12, p < .01$		$t = 0.07$, n.s.		$t = 1.52$, n.s.	

conditions were unintentionally worsened by inappropriate therapy.[4] These show a lowering of dissolved $CO_2 + H_2CO_3$ levels, with a consequent rise in plasma pH. The direction of these changes is in conformance with the hypothesis being suggested.

A cross-check on the interpretation advanced as to why certain nutrients aggravate the psychological conditions of Type I and Type II mentally ill *S*s is provided by a brief consideration of why other nutrients apparently improve the psychological conditions of some mentally ill *S*s.

It is being suggested that "fast oxidizing" Type II *S*s are metabolizing carbohydrates and glucogenic amino acids disproportionately faster than they are oxidizing fats and ketogenic amino acids, and that this differential utilization of carbohydrates appears to be related to their psychological state. Consequently, their mental and emotional symptoms would be worsened by factors that favor the increase of oxidation of such substrates, such as certain members of the B-complex vitamin group included in the Type I formula. However, since the opposite metabolic anomaly is hypothesized for the "slow oxidizing" Type I *S*s, the vitamins and minerals which worsen the psychological conditions of "fast oxidizers" might be expected to benefit the "slow oxidizers," if, among other factors, the carbohydrate metabolism is accelerated in one type and depressed in the other type.

This appears to be what happens. "Slow oxidizing" Type I *S*s whose average initial plasma level of dissolved $CO_2 + H_2CO_3$ before treatment was .73 mM/l showed an after-treatment value of 1.10 mM/l, an increase of approximately 50%, while at the start of treatment these *S*s had an average level of dissolved carbon dioxide plus carbonic acid which was 43% lower than for the "fast oxidizing" Type II group.

On the other hand, if Type II *S*s are utilizing carbohydrates and glucogenic amino acids more rapidly than they are fats and ketogenic amino acids, the substances which may tend to further the oxidation of fats in "slow oxidizing" Type I *S*s ought also to have the same effect in "fast oxidizing" Type II *S*s, resulting in a lowering of dissolved CO_2 levels with resultant increases in plasma pH and bicarbonate.

Again, this appears to be what occurs. At the beginning of the experiment the "fast oxidizing" Type II *S*s showed an average dissolved $CO_2 + H_2CO_3$ level of 1.27 mM/l, while at the end of the test this was reduced to 1.04 mM/l, a reduction of 22%. Since this reduction

[4] Date on these 4 *S*s were obtained in exploratory tests which preceded the experiment reported in this paper.

occurred at the same time there was a net increase in the level of total CO_2 (from 24.62 mM/l to 25.19 mM/l), it appears that the reduction in dissolved $CO_2 + H_2CO_3$ reflects an increase in the oxidation of fatty acids and ketogenic amino acids.

The following considerations appear to support such an interpretation. Table 2 presents the before-treatment differences between Type I and Type II *S*s in fasting total lipids and blood sugar. "Slow oxidizing" Type I *S*s reveal very significantly lower total lipid values and higher blood-sugar levels than do Type II "fast oxidizers," suggesting a differential utilization of fats rather than carbohydrates by Type I *S*s, while the reverse appears to occur in Type II *S*s.

Before and after treatment data on these variables for the whole experimental group are not available. However, values for 2 *S*s from whom before and after tests were obtained are given in Table 10. The

TABLE 10

BEFORE AND AFTER TREATMENT DIFFERENCES IN VENOUS PLASMA PH, BIBARBONATE, DISSOLVED CO_2 + H_2CO_3, FASTING TOTAL LIPIDS, AND FASTING BLOOD SUGAR IN TYPE I AND TYPE II MENTALLY ILL *S*s

Time	Plasma pH	Bicarbonate	Dissolved $CO_2+H_2CO_3$	Total Lipids	Blood Sugar
		Type I "Slow Oxidizing" *S*			
Before	7.50	17.50	.69	550	108
After	7.43	24.50	1.14	700	86
		Type II "Fast Oxidizing" *S*			
Before	7.36	23.50	1.29	1235	76
After	7.45	24.50	1.10	830	106

"slow oxidizing" Type I *S* (Subject 6, Tables 5 and 6) showed a full clinical remission of schizophrenic reaction of 10 years' duration at the same time the CO_2 content increased 40%, with a concomitant increase in blood lipids and decrease in blood sugar. This suggests that an increase in carbohydrate utilization occurred, resulting in increased energy production.

On the other hand, the "fast oxidizing" Type II *S* (Subject 4, Tables 5 and 7) showed a marked reduction in symptoms of anxiety and fatigue, permitting him to work for the first time in several years. Of interest here is an increase in fasting blood sugar with a concurrent reduction in total lipids and dissolved $CO_2 + H_2CO_3$, suggesting an increased utilization of fats as compared to carbohydrates. Of possible significance in this case is that *S*, prior to participating in this experiment, had been treated for hyperinsulinism on the basis of an abnormal glucose tolerance curve. This treatment was claimed by *S* to have been helpful, although the dietary management prescribed did not result in establishing a normal glucose tolerance curve. However, at the end of the test period his glucose tolerance was normal, which suggests that the apparent increase in oxidation of fats might be a factor in his increased energy, since an increase in the utilization of fats would tend to raise and to stabilize his blood-sugar level.

Conclusion

This study together with previous experiments (10, 12, 13) suggests that some cases of mental illness apparently may involve impairment of nervous system function due to abnormalities in intermediary metabolism. Normal cellular metabolic balance depends upon several factors, including an adequate supply of nutrients to provide both substrate as well as vitamins and minerals to participate in the synthesis of cellular enzymes, together with hormones such as thyroid and insulin which help regulate the rate of cellular oxidation.

Consequently, anomalies in intermediary metabolism may reflect many different conditions, such as inadequate food intake, poor digestion and assimilation, as well as endocrine disorders. In addition, both physical and emotional stress can disturb normal metabolic functions. Of interest in this connection is the observation that periods of intense psychological stress which several *S*s encountered during the course of the research here reported were found to result in decreases in the rates of oxidation in Type I "slow oxidizers," and increases in the rates of oxidation in Type II "fast oxidizers." This finding suggests that one important etiological factor in the disturbed intermediary metabolism of some of these mentally ill *S*s is psychological stress, which may increase the need for selective co-factors such as represented by the Types I and II vitamins and minerals for the respective types of *S*s.

One of the major difficulties confronting investigators in the field of biological psychiatry has been the failure to obtain a consistent set of deviations from normal values in blood variables in types of mental illness. Perhaps one of the reasons for this failure is suggested by the results of the present study, namely, that the clinical picture presented by one patient may be very similar to the clinical picture presented by another patient, but the identical symptom complex apparently can accompany entirely different biochemical anomalies. Conversely, such widely divergent clinical pictures as presented by obsessive-compulsive neurosis and periodic catatonia may each be accompanied by similar metabolic disturbances.

In view of these considerations, it appears desirable to supplement or supplant descriptive psychological criteria with a classificatory system based upon similarities and differences in metabolic profiles. Such an approach might help eliminate some of the confusion in research in mental illness, for it is obvious that if we group all "schizophrenics" together and simply average the result of measurements made on an apparently heterogeneous population, possible clues may be obscured by such treatment of the data.

There seems little doubt but that this kind of interpretation of experimental results is common and that it does in fact lead to confusion and controversy. Three examples may be cited.

Hoskins (5) in a study of oxygen consumption in 214 male schizophrenics reported finding an average rate of 88.3% of standard normal. However, an examination of the measurements upon which this average was based shows that the rates of individual patients varied from 55% of normal to 150% of normal, from being representative of what we have termed "slow oxidizers" to being "fast oxidizers." The author himself expresses doubt in his summary whether his results generally reflect "nosological homogeneity."

In another study of metabolism in schizophrenia by Kety, *et al.* (6), comparing 22 patients with normal controls, it is stated that "on the basis of these data a generalized change in circulation or oxygen utilization by the brain of schizophrenics may safely be ruled out. . . ." Cerebral oxygen consumption in schizophrenia is "identical" to that in normal healthy adults. A closer examination of the data upon which these conclusions are offered, however, shows a range of arterial blood pH from 7.30 to 7.50, with the range of dissolved $CO_2 + H_2CO_3$ extending from .72 mM/l to 1.48 mM/l.[5]

In terms of the language of the present study, 20 out of 22 of Kety's patients are what would have been classified as "fast oxidizers" had they participated in the research here reported. In other words, on the basis of the findings of the present study, Kety, *et al.* did not test a representative sample of the schizophrenic population. They appear to have all but missed the "slow oxidizers" and as a result have apparently reported the coincidence that their experimental group was "identical" to normal controls in brain metabolism.

Confirmation of this suggestion that Kety, *et al.* did not study a representative sample of schizophrenics is found in the contradictory re-

[5] These values for dissolved $CO_2 + H_2CO_3$ are not given in the original but were computed on the basis of the pH and the CO_2 content, which are given.

sults obtained by Gordon, *et al.* (4). In a study directed at confirming the results of Kety, Gordon tested cerebral oxygen uptake in 24 schizophrenics and found only one to be normal, 3 were above normal, while 21 were below normal. In terms of the present report, if Kety may have failed to include the "slow oxidizers," Gordon appears to have all but missed the "fast oxidizers." On the other hand, Hoskins appears to have found that the term schizophrenic does not signify a homogeneous population, metabolically.

That this is apparently so is illustrated in the study here reported, for 7 out of 11 schizophrenics were Type I "slow oxidizers," with an average plasma pH of 7.53, while 4 were Type II "fast oxidizers," with an average plasma pH of 7.35. However, if we had proceeded upon the assumption that the term "schizophrenic" signified a well-defined population from a biochemical point of view, we would have averaged these values and obtained a pH of 7.46 for the group, a value which some might interpret to be "normal." If such a "normal" value is now accepted as accurately characterizing the schizophrenic population, it will effectively hide a possibly vital clue, as well as acting to discourage further research in this particular area by other investigators.

REFERENCES

1. Brozek, J., & Erickson, N. K. Item analysis of the psychoneurotic scales of the Minnesota Multiphasic Personality Inventory in experimental semi-starvation. *J. Consult. Psychol.*, 1948, 12, 403–411.

2. Gambino, S. R. Normal values for adult human venous plasma pH and CO_2 content. *Tech. Bull. Registry Med. Technol.*, 1959, 29, 132–135.

3. Goldberger, E. *Water, electrolyte, and acid-base syndromes.* Philadelphia: Lea & Febiger, 1959.

4. Gordon, G. S., Estess, F. M., Adams, J. E., Bowman, K. M., & Simon, A. Cerebral oxygen uptake in chronic schizophrenic reaction. *A.M.A. Arch. Neurol. Psychiat.*, 1955, 73, 544–545.

5. Hoskins, R. G. Oxygen consumption ("basal metabolic rate") in schizophrenia. *Arch. Neurol. Psychiat.*, 1932, 28, 1346–1364.

6. Kety, S. S., Woodford, R. B., Harmel, M. H., Freyhan, F. A., Appel, K. E., & Schmidt, C. F. Cerebral blood flow and metabolism in schizophrenia. *Amer. J. Psychiat.*, 1948, 104, 765–770.

7. Keys, A., Brozek, J., Henschel, A., Mickelson, O., & Taylor, H. L. *The biology of human starvation.* Minneapolis: Univer. Minnesota Press, 1950.

8. Peterman, R. A., & Goodhart, R. S. Current status of vitamin therapy in nervous and mental disease. *J. Clin. Nutrit.*, 1954, 2, 11–21.

9. Richter, D. (Ed.) *Schizophrenia, somatic aspects.* New York: Pergamon, 1957.

10. Watson, G. Vitamin deficiencies in mental illness. *J. Psychol.*, 1957, 43, 47–63.

11. Watson, G. Note on nutrition in mental illness. *Psychol. Rep.*, 1960, 6, 202.

12. Watson, G., & Comrey, A. L. Nutritional replacement for mental illness. *J. Psychol.*, 1954, 38, 251–264.

13. Watson, G., & Currier, W. D. Intensive vitamin therapy in mental illness. *J. Psychol.*, 1960, 49, 67–81.

14. Wohl, M. G., & Goodhart, R. S. (Eds.) *Modern nutrition in health and disease.* Philadelphia: Lea & Febiger, 1960.

Acknowledgments

The author wishes to express his very deep gratitude to Prof. Andrew Comrey of the University of California at Los Angeles for his continuing advice and help in this research in matters of experimental design, analysis and presentation of data, in the preparation of the manuscript, and in many other ways, not the least of which has been his continuing support and encouragement. The author also acknowledges with deepest appreciation the medical and technical supervision of this research and the continuing aid and constant support provided by Dr. W. D. Currier, Medical Director of the Lancaster Foundation, without whose dedication and help the present study could not have been completed.